YOGA

FOR A

WORLD

OUT OF

BALANCE

To Louise,

Enjoy!

Also by Michael Stone

The Inner Tradition of Yoga:
A Guide to Yoga Philosophy for the Contemporary Practitioner

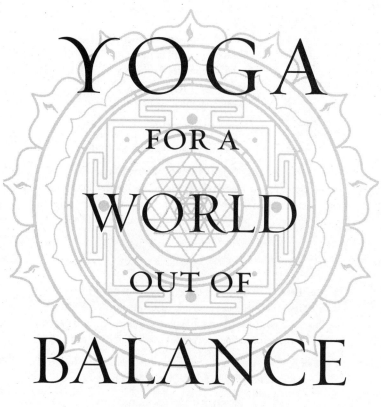

YOGA

FOR A

WORLD

OUT OF

BALANCE

Teachings on
Ethics and Social Action

MICHAEL STONE

SHAMBHALA
BOSTON & LONDON 2009

Shambhala Publications, Inc.
Horticultural Hall
300 Massachusetts Avenue
Boston, Massachusetts 02115
www.shambhala.com

© 2009 by Michael Stone

Page 207 constitutes a continuation of the copyright page.

9 8 7 6 5 4 3 2 1
First edition
Printed in Canada
♾ This edition is printed on acid-free paper that meets
the American National Standards Institute z39.48 Standard.
♻ This book was printed on 100% postconsumer recycled paper.
For more information please visit www.shambhala.com.

Distributed in the United States by Random House, Inc.,
and in Canada by Random House of Canada Ltd

Designed by DEDE CUMMINGS DESIGNS

Library of Congress Cataloging-in-Publication Data
Stone, Michael, 1974–
Yoga for a world out of balance: teachings on ethics and social action
/ Michael Stone
p. cm.
Includes bibliographical references.
ISBN 978-1-59030-705-2 (pbk.: alk. paper)
1. Yoga. I. Title
B132.Y6S7645 2009
181'.45—dc22
2009008426

We are all framed of flaps and patches and of so
shapeless and diverse a contexture that every
piece and every moment playeth its part.
—MONTAIGNE, *Essays*

Questions are better than answers.
—WALLACE STEVENS

Contents

A Note on Pronunciation
of Sanskrit Terms

I HAVE TRIED to keep technical terms to a minimum in this book although there are some Sanskrit terms for which there are no accurate English translations.

The transliteration of Sanskrit into English is always an approximation at best. The short *a* in Sanskrit is pronounced like the *u* in the English word "but," and the long *ā* is pronounced like the *a* in "father." In terms of the family of consonants, an easy approximation is possible by pronouncing *c* as in the *ch* in "church," *j* as in "jump," *s* as in the *sh* in "shut," *s* as in "sun," and *ś* as something halfway between the previous two. Aspirated consonants are quite distinct: *bh* as in "cab horse," *dh* as in "madhouse," *gh* as in "doghouse," *ph* as in "top hat," and *th* as in "goatherd." *R* is a vowel, pronounced somewhere between the *ri* in "rim" and the *er* in "mother." The transliterated letter and character *ñ* found in a word like *Patañjali* can be pronounced like the *ni* in "onion," and when found with the letter *j* as in the word *prajña,* can be pronounced like the *gn* in the word "igneous." Sometimes I pluralize a word like *yama* by simply adding an *s,* resulting in *yamas,* which is unacceptable for the academic or Sanskritist, but essential for simple reading for those unfamiliar with the language.

Unless otherwise attributed, the translations are my own. Try your best to pronounce these new sounds—as one gets used to them they open the palate and help concentrate the mind. Enjoy!

Foreword

I AM PRIVILEGED to read Michael Stone's book, *Yoga for a World Out of Balance: Teachings on Ethics and Social Action*. He emphasizes the importance of the five principles of the *yama*, which are the first basic teachings of the eight aspects of yoga, and which are designed for all of us to live peacefully in dignity and honor (*māna*).

The eight aspects *(aṣṭāṅga)* of yoga comprise a subjective art, science, and philosophy that covers the five layers of the human being: the anatomical, physiological, mental, intellectual, and spiritual bodies. They also balance the ecosystem and environment of the elements (earth, water, fire, air, ether) with yogic ethical principles. In this work, Michael Stone has clearly brought these principles of yoga to life.

These ethical principles sustain friendliness, compassion, and happiness in all of us. Michael shows how a person can develop the ability to bear unpleasant things and uphold truthfulness when he or she practices these principles.

If the individual is the world, the world is also the individual. One learns through yogic discipline the ways and means to balance one's life so that it's in rhythm with the environment around us. The flavor of yoga is that it helps us to interact and to express interrelationship by balancing not only within ourselves, but also in our relationships with one another and to our natural surroundings.

The five principles of yama are non-violence, truthfulness, non-misappropriation, chastity, and nonpossessiveness. These are considered by Patañjali to be universal ethical disciplines, to be followed by one and all, irrespective of race, gender, color, or climate.

For me, the term "yama" does not describe "self-restraint," as it is so often translated. Yama describes self-culture; as self-culture is universal, the ethical principles of the yama are therefore universal.

In India, Yama is considered to be the God of Death. Our instinctual nature includes the qualities of violence, dexterity instead of honesty, libertinism, greediness and the potential for stealing anything and everything, with no respect for our fellow beings. All these unethical desires, whether pursued directly or indirectly, cause death to the Self. Those who go against yama face imbalances, not only in their family but also within the society and community. These imbalances become the cause of death to the Self, even while the person remains alive. One who stays as much as possible with the principles of yama is bound to develop cleanliness and purity in body, mind, and speech.

Because Patañjali saw all the instinctual and intellectual defects that humans experience, he taught not only individual discipline through *niyama*, but also social discipline, through yama. Yama and niyama are expressed through external and internal cleanliness, contentment, passion to do good and to be good to one and all, control over body, mind, and speech, and resignation of all actions and their fruits to the divine.

Without morality, spirituality is out of the question. Michael Stone gives the example of Mahatma Gandhi, who followed the first two leaves, *ahimsā* and *satya*. I add Jina, Buddha, and Christ, who became immortals by adhering to Patañjali's principles of yama and niyama.

Michael Stone's book should be read by those who love to live in splendor and dignity. This Earth belongs to all of us. We are all one family here (*vasudhaiva kutumbam*). Michael Stone has written this book expressing the importance of yama and niyama for all on Earth to follow.

B. K. S. Iyengar
NOVEMBER 23, 2008
PUNE, INDIA

YOGA

FOR A

WORLD

OUT OF

BALANCE

INTRODUCTION

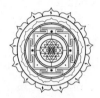

THE HUMAN WORLD is continually speeding up while the non-human world of plants, insects, and animals, with its once vast range of ecological diversity, is rapidly declining, causing irreversible imbalances throughout the web of life. A spiritual practice exclusively concerned with *my* enlightenment, *my* transcendence, or *my* emancipation from this life, this body, or this earth is not a spiritual practice tuned in to *these* times of ecological, social, physical, and psychological imbalance. The declining health of our ecosystems and the call for action in our cities, economies, communities, and families remind us that we don't have time to wait for enlightenment in isolated caves or inner sanctums; instead, it's time to consider action in the world and inner practice as synchronistic and parallel. Action in the world is not an externally imposed duty or simply a preliminary stage on the path to greater awareness but is in itself a valid spiritual path and an expression of interdependence, freedom, and awakening.

By seeing the inseparability of psychological change, ethical action, and spirituality, we can avoid the common fragmented and problematic view that spiritual practice takes us *away* from the world, thus excluding the body, householder life, and pressing contemporary issues like poverty, injustice, environmental degradation, or other forms of inequality and suffering. Yoga teaches us that everything is connected to everything else in the ongoing flux and flow of reality, beginning in the microcosm of the mind and extending all the way through the myriad forms of life. Yoga also claims freedom from suffering as its primary objective. It is from these realizations that our spiritual, ethical, and contemplative practices originate and mature. Wherever there is imbalance and suffering, yoga shows up.

Because of the sweeping changes of the modern era—including genetic research, the telephone, the Internet, high rates of literacy, swift air travel, two-column accounting systems, and faster and faster lifestyles—the Iron Age worldview out of which yoga teachings began to be described and refined can only offer us a partial platform, path, and set of truths. We begin in *this* culture at *this* time, so we must begin *now* to articulate and reenvision a yoga that is responsive to present circumstances—rooted in tradition yet adaptable and alive in contemporary times.

Yoga has always represented a radical path that leaves behind stiff metaphysics and doctrine and instead turns the practitioner's attention inward to the immediate experience of mind and body. The yogin studies the nature of reality as it presents itself here and now. As we turn toward the mind-body process, we begin to open to the temporary nature of our lives as well as the fact that we are inextricably woven into the very elements that constitute everything else—we *are* the natural world. For too long, yoga has been mischaracterized as an inner practice without understanding the teleology of practice. Yoga practices tune us in to reality by waking us up to the inherent transience of earthly life, the freedom that arises when wanting is relinquished, the truth that no thing is "me" or "mine," and the basic intelligence of the mind, body, and the life that supports us. The term "yoga" connotes the basic unity and interconnectedness of all of life including the elements, the breath, the body, and the mind. The techniques of yoga—including body practices, working with the breath, and discovering the natural ease of the mind—reorient practitioners to the very deep continuity that runs through every aspect of life until they realize that mind, body, and breath are situated in the world and not apart from worldly life in any way.

When I began practicing yoga, my primary focus was the physical practice of yoga postures, and every morning for the first six years I woke up to practice at five o'clock, six days a week. I sat in meditation for an hour, followed by standing postures, twists, forward bends, an hour of back bending and inversions, and finally breakfast. When I had any free time, I attended academic lectures on Indian philosophy, completed two degrees in psychology and religion, and studied Sanskrit; but the formality of my practice began to feel separate from the world I moved through, and I felt that formal practice and daily life had little in common. The connection between meditation, the physical practice of yoga, and the spiritual discipline to which it belonged became ambiguous and vague, and though I could intellectually grasp the connection between waking up the body and stilling the mind, I didn't understand how to put these practices into action in everyday life. While I was having significant insights in meditative practices, I felt formal practice and daily life were not seamlessly interwoven.

This is true for many contemporary yoga practitioners, and as I now teach extensively, the most common question I hear is how to integrate philosophy, body practices, meditation, and daily life together with our role in relationships, concerns about the world around us, and the desire to take action in a world out of balance. Even when students begin having genuine experiences of insight or meditative quietude, I always ask them how they are going to incorporate these experiences into their daily activities. How does spiritual practice support and motivate our choices and ambitions? How can my personal enlightenment be the goal of practice if there is so much suffering around me? If the domain of any spiritual tradition is the relief and transformation of suffering, what does yoga, one of the great spiritual traditions, have to say about contemporary forms of suffering and existential disorientation?

For the practitioner of hatha yoga—the meditative practice of waking up to present experience in mind and body—the link between yoga as a "practice" and a "spirituality" is often realized through an intuition rather than through intellectual articulation. However, intuition is not enough; nor is it enough to imagine that yoga offers a complete set of codes or truths that can, like mathematical equations, tell us what to do in every given situation. The world is too complex, too nuanced, and it's always shifting. Therefore, we need to investigate the practical ways that yoga practice matures both in formal study and in everyday life. Today, our personal, ecological, and social situations present unique and direct challenges to every one of us to respond to the great existential questions of life and death, to look deeply into interdependence, and to fully actualize our awakening in a world distressed and in need. How is our awakening going to contribute to the world at large? Why is our spiritual path important for the great rivers, the butterflies, and the architecture of our cities?

BEGINNING WITH MIND AND BODY

Since the exploration of your physical being involves focusing and settling the reactionary patterns of the mind, and since settling the mind opens each of us up to a much wider spectrum of reality, the interdependence of the mind and body become the main thrust of yoga as a spiritual path. In fact, since the body is always present, the body is where we begin. But what is the body exactly? Is the body simply a collection of bones and skin and mental activities? Where does the body begin and end?

If my body is made primarily of water and animated by the breath, is it possible to call the water in the body "mine" and the air outside of my lungs "the world"? When I pay close attention to the workings of the body, I'm taken immediately into the mind and the ways in which I perceive and feel the body. Furthermore, I notice that the body can't be separated from the natural world except in my imagination, and so it becomes hard to talk about a body practice as separate from a world practice. I move the body and I'm moving a corner of the world;

I sweep the floor with attentiveness and I sweep my mind. "As realization dawns," Patañjali states, even "the distinction between breathing in and breathing out falls way."[1] I settle into the accordion-like movements of the inhalation and exhalation and, over time, the elaborations of the mind quiet down and I actually *become* the breath—a body breathing the world; the world breathing in this very body. Who is breathing whom?

Like most spiritual practices, the aim of yoga is not perfect mastery over technique or the ability to memorize scriptures, but rather the activity of bringing one's insights and sensitivities into the world through action. Through the release of habitual patterns of attachment and reactivity, we are better able to perceive and take action in the world. When I tune in to the fact that the body and world are in deep continuity with one another, when I stand up after formal practice and look into the smoggy skyline, I feel called to take action. Yoga occurs when our inner work manifests in the world around us.

The world of mind and body, in the nondual tradition of yoga, is inseparable from the larger world of the birdsong, towering pines in old-growth groves, slow and aging rivers, industrial exhaust, or the crystal clear eyes of a newborn human. The interconnected reality we call "yoga" orients us toward a mode of perception that sees reality as an interconnected web in which our own small story line is only a part and certainly not the most prominent.

SPIRITUALITY AND ECOLOGICAL IMBALANCE

We are living in times of unrestraint. That we have caused immeasurable and irreversible damage to the human and nonhuman world has pressed many thinkers, teachers, and activists, therapists, seekers, and scientists to consider not simply how this objectification of the world came to be but what we can do about it. The world's spiritual traditions are confronted with an ecological crisis and existentially confused populations. It is to these issues that all spiritual traditions must respond if they are to serve the goals of freedom, happiness, and compassion that they promise. These goals can't be served by reinventing ideologies or theological viewpoints. We must tune in to the rivers, to one another, to the vinegar fog that surrounds every city. It is in this troubled world that we practice yoga, and it is to this reality that we must respond.

What informs the choices we make? How do people change? What is the relationship between restraint and action? How do we practice restraint and renunciation in a secular and consumer-driven culture without falling into dogmatic codes or idealistic commandments? What role do ethics play in psychological change, and why have ethics always been the guiding principle of religious activity? How do cultures change, and why is the current response to economic injustice, environmental damage, interpersonal violence and war so slow, especially in countries where our creative capacities and helping abilities are so powerful? Where do our spiritual beliefs and practices intertwine with personal, social, and ecological responsibility?

This book is a response to these questions. In these times of overconsumption, overproduction, and massive gaps of inequality among economies and families, and also among ecological systems, it's time to think about the psychological dimensions of change.

CHANGING OUR MINDS

Looking deeply into change begins by meditating on the effect of our actions, studying how we organize our experience and, as an end point, becoming increasingly sensitive to all life including the lives of fish, buildings, and highways. Most of our individual and global ills have been brought on by a culture unrestrained by the greater human and nonhuman good, and spiritual practice has always been characterized as tuning in to something other than our endless desires and wants. Change and sensitivity begin with how we make choices, and how we make choices begins with our psychology. "Psychology" refers to the way we organize our experience based on the interaction of present circumstances and the momentum of our habit energies. Habit energies are the psychological, physiological, cultural, and ancestral patterns that inform how we perceive, think, and make choices moment to moment. They are primarily outside of our awareness. It is through our mind-body process that we perceive the world and through this same process that we can effect change.

It's easy to conceptualize the relationship between humans and the world as separate, but when we look clearly and sincerely, we find ourselves enmeshed and completely embedded in the living form we call life. When we perceive the world as mechanistic, as independent from "me," and as some "thing" that is manipulatable, we act out of dualistic assumptions. Creating separateness in a world not inherently separate is like trying to conceive of human beings unlinked to the world around us. When we perceive life in such a self-centered way, our grammar and viewpoint follow: I wake up as *my*self, work to acquire *my* food for *my* family, and put *my* money in *my* bank account for *my* future, for *my* lifetime.

If we *are* our own lives—expressions of the natural world breathing itself—there is no need to think of transcendence as taking us anywhere other than here. The ground of yoga begins with *this* ground—a nurturing source that is not hidden or waiting for us in a future lifetime. Any ground we look at is much like water—always changing and flowing—but just like water, it does not have to be solid to nurture us.

There is nowhere else to go; this is it, and there is no way to enhance the quality of our lives and those around us if we believe that the goal of spiritual practice is to get beyond the body, the earth, and the vicissitudes of everyday life. How can we generate a life of love and devotion if we value an idealized life beyond this one as the goal of practice? How can we care for the earth if we don't live with an immediate connection to the body, the life of the mind, and the natural world? In *Mind in Life,* Evan Thompson writes:

We can travel a path from life to consciousness to intersubjectivity and culture that can do justice to our existence as living bodily subjects. The individual human subject is the enculturated bodily subject. In this way, the knowing and feeling subject is not the brain in the head, or even the brain plus the body, but the socially and culturally situated person, the enculturated human being.[2]

We are made of our ancestry—earth, air, water, and all of the elements—and yet, when we deny these origins, we turn those elements into commodities rather than resources. We measure water in terms of its exportability, forests in terms of their board feet, and land in terms of real estate value. Through unethical business practices, people have become "consumers" and communities are categorized as "markets" or "sectors." At a psychological level, the self is also commodified when it is treated as an object to be improved, perfected, or worshipped. When the self is reified and restricted to an image of our own making, we take flight from the totality of our interdependence. It is through the realization that the self is just another element of life—contingent and provisional—that we can take action no longer dominated by self-concern, self-doubt, or self-aggrandizement. This is nondualism: the structural foundation of an authentic life characterized by ethical responsibility, intimacy, meaning, and compassion.

Two things need to change. First, we need to understand the causal relationship between our actions and the effects of our actions. Second, once sensitive to the devastating effect of our actions in the human and nonhuman world, we need practical skills for learning how to take action, especially when our minds are caught up in reactivity and distraction and are unable to touch the present moment. From there, we can begin to plant positive seeds in the mind, body, and body politic.

Action begins in our present circumstances. In our distracted, busy, entertainment-driven culture, it is not only hard to slow down but also to pay attention to that which is outside of our preferences and expectations. It is difficult to be present from moment to moment in this attention-deficit society.

Being distracted and caught in habitual patterns of addiction and aversion leads to a life of alienation and apathy. It becomes hard to find a center. A center, in this case, connotes sensitivity to our own body and the body of the world, to our own mind and the minds of others, and to the effects of our speech both internally and externally. Lost in self-judgment, guilt, blame, anxiety, or depression, it becomes hard to take in a world outside of our own thoughts and feelings. Not receiving and responding to a world beyond these limiting symptoms reinforces those very symptoms and cuts us off from others and ourselves.

Since we are in a shared existence with the human world, the non-human natural world, and the human-built world, we need to suspend some of our reactivity and distraction to look anew at what is actually happening in our own minds, bodies, families, and all relations, extending all the way from our own thoughts to the vast sky witnessing the experience of all of us. Environmental or social action must be accompanied by skills that help us practice stillness and compassion; otherwise our anger or irritation may get the better of us. Without such clarity, we don't know how to settle our lives and tend to the great questions that being alive presents to us.

Psychological change then is intimately related to spirituality because when we change to become more open, flexible, patient, and sensitive, we open to a world greater than the frosted and hemmed-in world of our thoughts. When we open to a greater world, we open to the greater good; spiritual awakening then becomes a process of cultural and ecological awakening. Spiritual change, psychological change, and ethical action go hand in hand, forming together an interconnected path of awakening. Awakening to what? Awakening to the effect of our actions, the importance of individual and social change, and sensitivity to a world beyond "me" that occurs when we can find the place in us that is deeper than our opinions. Change begins in the present moment.

Spiritual life and contemplative practice always happen within a world of living beings, and therefore nothing can be excluded from the range our practice. Every aspect of the web of life has a part to play in the greater system of ecological existence. Part of our responsibility as human beings is to live in a sustainable and respectful way among all of the biota, elements, emotions, and energies that contribute to and sustain the integral balance of life. This book begins by describing how yoga teachings on causality and renunciation give rise to intimacy and ethics. The mind, body, and body politic are inseparable.

The central five sections of the book each deal with the five ethical principles described in the *Yoga-Sūtra* attributed to Patañjali. These principles are called "yama," which literally means "restraint," and include nonharming (ahimsā), honesty (satya), nonstealing (asteya), the wise use of energy (brahmacarya), and nonacquisitiveness (aparigrahā). Within each chapter there are diversions and examples, definitions and commentaries; you can read the text in a linear way or move through chapters that speak to where you are at in your own life. Whatever route you choose through the text, the terms will become clear and the teachings cumulative as each yama loops back into the others, forming a kind of web without beginning or end. The web is held together by the teachings of karma (causality) and samādhi (integration)—two terms that appear as consistent themes throughout each chapter.

Like the yamas themselves, the chapters flow out of one another and then loop back through each other, though they all stem from the profound link between insight into interconnectedness and action rooted in nonviolence. In an age where many of us struggle to find clarity in our approach to spirituality as well as the most helpful forms of action in a world out of balance, these chapters and principles may offer some guidance.

CHAPTER ONE

THE PATH UNFOLDS

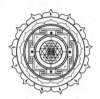

I N O R D E R T O investigate the psychological and spiritual dimensions of our current global ills, it's important to look back at ancient
models of practice, change, and wisdom that may be of benefit to us
now. Perhaps there is something our eager culture has forgotten in its
rush forward. We look back not idealistically but rather with openness
to what another culture at another time may have to teach us about our
minds, bodies and place in the world, even though this ancient wisdom must be brought to life in an entirely different cultural context.
Looking back at seminal texts like the *Yoga-Sūtra* also might inspire us
to see how other yogins responded to the cultural imbalances of their
particular time. Some initial contact with the insights offered by Patañjali, the reputed author of the *Yoga-Sūtra*, may better equip us to put
yoga to work on contemporary issues and see if we might begin to learn
something from an ancient wisdom tradition struggling to come to life
in contemporary culture.

Some time between the third century B.C.E. and the turn of that
millennium, only four centuries after the dharma teachings of Siddhar-
tha Gautama Buddha, prior to the birth of Jesus, just after the Great
Wall of China was constructed, and sometime around the assassination of Julius Caesar, a mythological sage named Patañjali codified the
practice of yoga somewhere in northern India. Nothing is known about

Patañjali other than an intuited sense of a person deeply committed to meditation practice, teaching, and integrating diverse teachings of the time.

The term *sūtra* is a predecessor of the English word "suture" and refers to the precise tying together of previously disparate philosophies and practices. Sūtra form, concise and dense philosophical verse, exists in all schools of Indian philosophy where great teachers or communities attempted to codify, in the most precise way, the scheme and path of their spiritual practice. Practice could involve anything from techniques of breathing or hand placement in postures to dialectical arguments concerning the nature of the mind or precise descriptions of stages of meditation and even ethics. Patañjali's *Yoga-Sūtra* is considered one of the seminal texts of the yoga tradition because it covers all these bases and borrows from the most unexpected places, including Saṃkhya Yoga and the Buddhadharma.

Patañjali's *Yoga-Sūtra* is best known for articulating the royal path of yoga (raja yoga) by describing eight interrelated limbs of practice known as aṣṭāṅga yoga ("aṣṭā" means eight; "aṅga" is a limb), the eight-limbed path of yoga. Beginning with restraints and ethics (yama), the eight limbs are as follows:

1. Yama (external restraint): the clarification of one's relationship to the human and nonhuman world

2. Niyama (internal restraint): personal principles governing the cultivation of insight, including śauca (purification), santoṣha (contentment), tapas (discipline, patience), svādhyāya (self-study, contemplation), and īśavara-pranidhāna (devotion, aspiration, and dedication to the ideal of pure awareness)

3. Āsana (posture): cultivation of profound physical and psychological steadiness and ease in mind, breath, and body; practice of yoga postures

4. Prāṇāyāma (breath and energetic regulation): sustained observation and relaxation of all aspects of breathing, bringing about a natural

refinement of the mind-body process through the stilling of the respiratory process

5. Pratyāhāra (uncoupling of the senses): a naturally occurring uncoupling of sense organs from sense objects as awareness becomes interiorized

6. Dhāraṇā (concentration meditation): locking awareness on a single object (for example, sound, breath, or sensations in body) until the field of awareness becomes singular and focused

7. Dhyāna (absorption): concentration deepens to the point where subject and object dissolve and the sense of "me" is temporarily absent

8. Samādhi (integration): the sustained experience of concentration where there is a complete integration of subject and object, revealing pure awareness and interconnectedness

Whenever I begin working with students who want to establish a well-rounded practice, we always begin with the first limb of practice, the yamas, as a means of setting a foundation for what spiritual practice means and how it ripens in contemporary life. This approach helps dismantle our lofty associations with the term "spiritual" so that practice begins grounded in the material. When we begin with the five yamas, our yoga practice grows roots in the intricate and infinite web of living relationships and thus presses the yoga practitioner not to turn away from the world but to tune in to and be tuned by the life of relational existence. How we relate to ourselves, other humans, plants, animals, architecture, city planning, the growing of food, and the daily tasks in the household is part and parcel of the path of yoga practice. Sometimes people are not sure how to begin a practice and even how to mature a practice once they've begun. This list is not just sequential but gives us an overview of the varied elements that constitute a path. Although we use these lists as suggestions, how they manifest in a unique life looks very different for each individual and community.

The first limb, yama, is comprised of five guidelines designed to clarify our relationship to the human, nonhuman, and human-built worlds.

1. Ahiṃsā: not harming, nonviolence, not having the intention to cause injury
2. Satya: honesty, being truthful
3. Asteya: not taking what is not freely given, not stealing
4. Brahmacarya: wise use of energy, including sexual energy
5. Aparigrahā: not being acquisitive, not being greedy, not accumulating what is not essential

Indian philosophers cherished lists. We've been handed lists of obstacles, lists of factors to awakening, five factors that cause suffering, five sheaths of mind and body, seventy-two thousand nadis listed in great detail and placed on the fifty-one petals called chakras. Lists and more lists permeate ancient texts. However, the five yamas are not categorized phenomena or sacred lists; instead, they are suggestions for what to do and how to take action both in stillness and in the frenzy and paradox of daily life. "The yamas are not what you *should not* do," a teacher once told me, "but what you *should* do." The yamas are practical; there is nothing holy in their practice.

Patañjali is often depicted as having a serpent's tail with human arms and a human face. Patañjali's form as both serpent and human—a double image we find in many mythological genres and systems—represents the theoretical and the practical, the idealist and the realist, the spiritual and the utilitarian. Without practice, theory is superficial; without critical engagement with traditional teachings and texts, practice can be misguided. Patañjali may embody the truth of an enlightened being, one free from discontent, but he also bears a common human face like you and I. His text is practical, not holy.

The word "text" is related to the Latin word for "weave." To be faithful to a text, especially an ancient text that has been studied, practiced, and commented upon for at least two thousand years, we have to weave it into the fabric of our daily lives so that it comes alive and is not just something of antiquarian interest.

The yamas help us understand and refine our behavior. As we watch our own ecology—how it connects, disconnects, inhales and exhales, falls apart, rights itself—we come to see a life that exists in a much wider field than the purely personal.

LEAVING NOTHING OUT

Yoga is the reality of leaving nothing out. We all have an imperative not to place fish outside the realm of moving waters, nor should we place clouds, the atmosphere, mountains, human relationship, or thought anywhere outside of our own personal being. And what constitutes "personal" being if I do not separate myself out of the interdependent flow and web of life itself? If I am nothing other than that which I perceive, if I am nothing other than frogs and stars and trees, how can I place myself at the center of the universe? How can I create an effective environmental stance if I keep putting myself in the center, looking out at a world that surrounds me?

A dualistic approach to ecology does not work if it places the human being in objective relation to the world and not of it. Nondualism, in a spiritual and ecological sense, proposes a radical challenge to the presumption that humans have dominance over nature. Western scientific rationality has created a view of the nonhuman world as dead and therefore materially, politically, and economically available for exploitation. But nature *is* yoga: relational, interdependent, united, holistic, and nonhierarchical. Even humanity must be seen in all its manifestations as nature in its widest sense, otherwise we remain caught in a mechanistic view of nature as entirely separate from the human being. The mechanistic view that we have inherited from the sixteenth century imagines nature as mechanistic, whereby nature has no inherent purpose and simply follows the mechanical laws that govern matter in motion. René Descartes played a key role in this mechanistic view by claiming that mind, nature, consciousness, and life are not only governed by observable mechanical laws, but that they are absolutely separate from one another. If consciousness and the living body are entirely separate, it's a quick step to thinking that the life of the body and the functioning of the natural world do not happen in tandem.

Patañjali sees life in a holistic way. Life is not outside of human form, and the forms things take are the essence of life itself. We are united with all things at all times. Everything is complete. Although at a superficial glance such a statement may seem like pure idealism or even passivity, it is exactly the opposite. It is *because* I recognize my part in the interconnectedness of reality that I begin to see that I have to take action. And since all of my actions have an effect, I need to pay attention to the kind of effect I want to have in the world—not just for my benefit but for the benefit of sentient and nonsentient existence, because it's only the human mind that creates the notion of separation. Or, turned around the other way, we could say that my response to the world is a way of learning how to live and what it is to live a life that is meaningful and responsive. Raising our children is raising ourselves; growing our gardens, we grow one another.

INTIMATE ACTIONS

Here is the mythological Patañjali, a serpent stretching from tail to shoulders with a human face looking out into the world. This image is a paradox of form: the stainless tail representing the nondual reality we call yoga and her head, a manifestation or expression of one's awakening in the always imperfect culture of humans.[1]

Being enlightened does not mean that one day you wake up and see the light. Being enlightened means that as you wake up more and more, you become sensitive to the world around and within you, developing an intimacy that contracting around self always destroys. Living from this unself-conscious place means being active and alive in the world without being enslaved by worldly identification. This is not *other*-worldly but *this*-worldly, not far away in some utopia but right here, in this body, in this mind, at this time. Waking up to the world, feeling yourself as only a part of it, and loving the interpenetrating parts that make up all of life is the goal and gradual fruition of spiritual practice.

In an ever-changing and deeply evanescent world, spiritual awakening offers us the end of a life organized by fear, isolation, and meaninglessness. Being cut off from relational existence through the creation of a "separate me" creates alienation and encloses us in a lonely carapace of self. A self that is cut off from the pulse of life is a self unmotivated, insensitive, and self-absorbed. Likewise, a culture cut off from the effects of its actions and ignorant of the mesh of "interpermeating" webs that create and sustain life is a culture without deep ethical commitments. A culture uninvolved and unaware of its background in relational existence is a society depressed. Human and collective psychology work in just the same ways: both begin with perception. If I perceive everything in terms of a "me" and "mine," the world will seem objective, at odds with, and alternately for or against me. Honoring each principle of life begins with a commitment to a life greater than self-reference and lifts us out of cultural malaise.

The English word "nature" is derived from the Latin *natura,* meaning "birth" or "constitution." This in turn is further derived from the root *nat,* which is where we get the words "native," "nation," and "natal." The natural wilderness and function of one's own mind and body are not distinct from the great fir forests, the ocean currents, or the current of breath streaming through the nostrils as you read these words. The belly expands when we inhale and softens as we exhale, and the mental world turns on the movements of these breaths. The mind is supported by the air we breathe, and the quality of the air is, in part, influenced by our actions in an endless cycle. Twelve billion years of DNA is animated in each and every breath cycle, moment after moment, season after season, lifetime after lifetime. "Although poverty and climate change seem unrelated," writes Paul Hawken in *Blessed Unrest,* "they have common roots for the simple reason that we are nature, literally, in every molecule and neuron."[2] When we are caught up in negative states of mind and self-reference, all of nature becomes objectified and exploited and seen in terms separate from our basic functioning.

The ordinary world, like the place of the body in spiritual life, should not be denied. It is the place of devotion and practice because it is always present and is the closest aspect of nature that we can study. Paul Hawken continues his description of the inseparability of the designations "human" and "nature":

> We contain clay, minerals, and water, are powered by sunshine through plant life, and are intricately bound to all other species, from fungi to marsupials to bacteria. In our lungs are oxygen molecules breathed by every type of creature ever to have lived on earth, along with the very hydrogen and oxygen atoms that Jesus, Confucius, and Rachel Carson breathed.[3]

The term "nature" connotes vastness because it leaves nothing out. Our yoga should be practiced this way also. "Then," Patañjali declares, "one is no longer disturbed by the play of opposites."[4]

I will always observe the heron from outside its world. I cannot know what it feels like to be a microorganism buried under twenty thousand years of ocean coral and algae, or a melting iceberg in the North Atlantic. But in the space I give to see these different elements of life moving, acting, living, and being, I create space in myself to perceive beyond the limits of preference, outside my world of likes and dislikes. Only then, when the mind and body are quiet enough, engaged enough, less reactive, can I begin to take in what is other. The more I can take in what is other, the less I need to construct a separate self, and the interconnectedness of life begins to impact my very nature. "Other" becomes a less useful, or skillful, category. How do you define the other? Who is the other? The mystical experience that comes from psychological change requires a next step: We need to act out of the awareness that "the other" is no other than you and I.

Sometimes we consider spiritual practice a technology devoted to having an elevated experience, be it oneness, openness, connectedness. However, once that experience ends, since it too is fleeting, we need to use the insights we've had to inform our actions. Once I see that I am nothing other than the parent with whom I argue, the dog I always yell at, or the tree I recently cut down, I need to follow my insight through with ethical action. Otherwise, spirituality becomes a passive philosophical stance that leads to nihilistic idealism.

Spiritual experience turns out to be another form of materialism when we find pleasure in spiritual insight or psychological change without continuing the work of waking up, which is gradual and context dependent. Each situation is brand new and requires a wise and spontaneous response; we can't just superimpose our spiritual philosophy across the board. Even when we are anchored in the breath, we come to see that the breath too is changing, that the anchor is shifting. If we only take action to feel good, the possibility of awakening remains limited, because it revolves around a "me" that needs to feel good. Experiences can be sudden, but the work of a committed spiritual practice is slow and circular. *Our insights need to be tested out in order for them to become sources of wisdom; otherwise we can rest in our insights and move slowly back into states of unconscious apathy, ideology, or unawareness.*

Patañjali teaches a path of freedom. What is inclusive about his teachings is that waking up *includes* the world rather than departing from it and that letting go of all forms of clinging, most especially clinging to a separate self, is the basis of spiritual life. The observation of rules and rituals is not a significant feature of Patañjali's method, nor would it be correct to say he had a unifying method at all. Patañjali's yoga culminates in waking up to the reality of an interconnected existence where the world moves transparently through us and where we take action without clinging, always moving deeper and deeper into the world without being caught in the mirage of self-image. Awakening without ethical action is only partial enlightenment; when the beasts of real war head home, when we find utter violence within ourselves, our communities, and families, and when we are no longer drunk on shopping, what are we to do?

DISTRACTED BY "I," "ME," AND "MINE"

All things exist from moment to moment. In the moment that something comes to be, it is as it is. Then it passes away. When we pay attention to the birth, aging, and death of life, we come to see that there is no thing we can hold on to anyway. How many thoughts have you had today? How many feelings have you had this week? How many sensations have you felt this hour? And where do they go? Where do thoughts and feelings come from?

We have no answers for these questions, because the sheer truth of change is stunning. It may be easy to let go of our contraction around some light thoughts or simple feelings, yet something seems to remain that is most difficult to release, namely, the ongoing, felt sense of a separate "me." "Clinging to self is habitual," says Patañjali in the third chapter of the *Yoga-Sūtra*, "even for the wise."[5]

In this way Patañjali clears the way for a profound path of awakening based on insight into the nature of self and eventually allowing that self to dissolve in the midst of the greater world, since the self *is* the world and not apart from it. It's the entanglement in our stories of "I," "me," and "mine" that keep us alienated from the flow of life, from ease, from intimacy. Spiritual practice is one of opening to something greater than the world of "me" and, as such, requires practices, guidelines, and encouragement for living a life beyond habits and personal preferences. As such, psychological change, for Patañjali, is inextricably tied with relationship and ethics. In fact, the eight limbs of yoga, for which he is so famous, always return the practitioner to a life grounded in action and relationship. The student on the path of yoga begins moving through life with greater care and decisiveness, growing into the world like countless buds on a branch, ordinary yet singular.

How you treat animals, how you grow your food, how you manage your resources internally and externally—these are all valid aspects of your yoga path because such actions form your very self. In fact, the choices you make in decisions that range from abortion to same-sex marriage, eating fish or growing corn, paving new highways or determining foreign policy, all form the basis of the yamas, the first limb of Patañjali's path of yoga. The first limb of yoga is your very own limb, your small intestine, your lungs, your very air.

CHAPTER TWO

RESTRAINT
IN TIMES OF
UNRESTRAINT

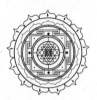

T HE WORLD DOES not exist for us; the world just exists. To say
that it is *for* us or *not for* us creates a fragmentation from the
outset that obscures the deep continuity of all life-forms and gives us a
false sense of separateness—an artificial division that yoga teachings try
to break through. The inherent union of all life—what we have defined
as "yoga"—is never beyond morality, because it's up to each of us to
express this union through all of our actions of body, speech, and mind.
We don't practice nonviolence as much as we *are* nonviolence; we don't
try to act compassionately—we actually *become* compassion. Whatever
is happening in the hearts and mind of others is also happening to us.
Whatever harm we cause to the rivers and rain clouds we also bring
upon ourselves; or are we defining our "selves" too narrowly? Reverence
for life begins when we realize that we are a microcosm of this vast continuity we call existence.

Human beings are not the most important life-form in the ecological matrix, but surely we have caused the most devastation to our
known ecological world. The richest 20 percent of the world's popula-

tion now receives 150 times the income of the poorest 20 percent.[1] The richest one-fifth of the world

- consumes 45 percent of all meat and fish, the poorest fifth 5 percent;
- consumes 58 percent of total energy, the poorest fifth less than 4 percent;
- has 74 percent of all telephone lines, the poorest fifth 1.5 percent;
- consumes 84 percent of all paper, the poorest fifth 1.1 percent;
- owns 87 percent of the world's vehicles, the poorest fifth less than 1 percent.[2]

Almost 800 million people—about one-sixth of the population of the world's developing nations—are malnourished. Two hundred million of them are children.[3] It is estimated that 880 million people lack access to basic health care and 1.3 billion lack access to safe drinking water. Seventeen million people die each year from curable diseases, including diarrhea, malaria, and tuberculosis. Five million of these people die due to water contamination.[4]

We live in times of unrestraint. Within a one-mile radius of my home in a Canadian city, I can purchase, even in the middle of a snowy winter, olives from Crete, organic spinach from California, garlic from China, a cashmere scarf from India, and a bottle of wine from just about anywhere; I can order products through the Internet or listen to radio on any international bandwidth. Our neighbors, refugees from Tibet, can hardly afford any of the aforementioned items, although their family dinner tonight, the gas that runs through their stove, the entertainment on the television that's playing as they cook, and the bottled water on the table will not be sourced locally. It's hard to wrap our minds around the way transportation patterns, digestion patterns, pollution, consumption, even the dinner table itself, impact the web we call life. Without attention to such connections, choices become life-destroying rather than life-affirming.

My bicycle was built in Sweden, our son's toys in Germany, our maple kitchen counter in Michigan, and I have no idea where our cat was born. Although much of our contemporary progress and change offers us significant improvement in the quality of our lives, that progress also hides a shadow. Karma reveals that shadow: the effects of our actions internally and externally. We most often think of karma as personal or something "spiritual" and not of the "material." Although the root *kr* of the word "karma" means "to do" or "to create," karma is not something you do or try to manipulate—it is something you *are* in every mode of your being. You *are* the choices you make.

Our dominant philosophy is one of unlimited material growth in all its manifestations: economic, industrial, reproductive. Even personal forms of growth like self-improvement projects and self-help groups are manifestations of individual and collective discontent that seeks to find happiness in anthropocentric ways. In this context, restraint seems, on the surface anyway, illogical: If we can have whatever we want whenever we want, why would we contemplate or even investigate the notion of restraint?

If we can't have what we want, we at least have the means to overproduce. We are a culture caught in a cycle of overconsumption and overproduction to meet our exponentially rising desire for more. If we don't have enough electricity to meet our needs, we can build another power plant. In fact, since our family lives on the lower end of the income scale, our federal government recently sent us a check to cover the costs of rising electricity bills. Although we receive money to pay our bills, the government doesn't ask us to restrain from using as much power as we do, nor do we hear from the government about limiting the ways we use electricity; instead we use the taxpayers' money to maintain a lifestyle so rarely questioned. Yet the economy, the environment, the mind, and the family must all be healthy for the others to survive—there is no dichotomy in such an equation. If we only think in terms of economic growth and if we are always motivated by the insatiable ghosts of endless desire, how do we measure the end point?

The course of spiritual practice found in the nondualistic traditions of Yoga, Buddhism, and Taoism offers us an understanding of and insight into the relational nature of reality and the interconnectedness of all things. Like many traditions, the Yoga tradition of Patañjali, a system known for its meditative practices, begins with a sophisticated understanding of relationship, interconnectedness, personal transformation, and ethics. Or, we might say the system is so very simple and basic to our nature. Even though the body is supported by and created of the natural world, the distracted and overly conceptual mind might be operating in an entirely different metaphor that is totally disembodied, heads and shoulders away from soil and rivers and rich night skies. In Patañjali's *Yoga-Sūtra*, there seems little or no difference between personal and collective transformation; as one deeply penetrates the first step of practice, the yamas—ethical principles that help guide us in our actions of body, speech, and mind—we have some guidelines as to how we can gear our choices to be in line with the wisdom that everything is interwoven.

A common question along these lines becomes: Why not just pay attention to our activities on the meditation cushion? Won't that bring about necessary changes? If I find stillness in my mind, doesn't that offer a positive contribution to the world at large? A good question to be certain, but such formal activities are only a part of practice, because eventually you will have to defecate, change your socks, source buckwheat for that little cushion, and the cushion may not help when you need to find firewood. Yoga is always a practice that takes place in the world, and so it makes no sense to deny your activities in the world, because that is the fabric of practice, the warp and weave of your life.

This valid and challenging question is actually a reminder that we need to meditate on the effect of our actions both individually and collectively and on the psychology behind our intentions and habits. While it's certainly true that intentions can be preconceptions that might be distracting at times, intentions are a tool we use to reorient the mind when we are caught in distracted or greedy states of mind. No matter, there is no escape from decision making and action. No book, system, or theory is ever going to offer us a specific guideline for what to do or how to live that will magically cut through the complexity of our unique situations. As I write these words from a deck in Los Angeles, I overhear news reports describing how the city water supply is full of pharmaceuticals that treatment plants have no way of breaking down. Viagra, Prozac, and numerous antibiotics do not break down after being evacuated from the human body. These chemicals and microorganisms move through the waterways with effects researchers are only beginning to study. All water comes together.

What kind of actions should one take in this situation? Obviously these kinds of decisions, which lie at the heart of our ideas about ourselves and nature, cannot be explored simply with Ten Commandments. Nor can any theory claim to be a universal canopy that covers all of the different norms and values across cultures, because doing good is always relative. Intentions and precepts, like any vow or commitment, can be broken a thousand times a day, but if you didn't set them out in the first place, you would never be able to imagine the better world they imply. While we cannot create an everlasting, universal theory of action or ethics, what we can do is offer an outline of the psychology of ethics. This is not to say that there is one universal psychology—because of course psychology always includes culture—but rather to begin to understand how most of our personal, ecological, and cultural ills are, at the base, problems of perception. The wise elder Bhisma instructs his younger nephew Yudhishthira on how to *become* peace:

> Even the gods are bewildered at the path
> Of the one who seeks the abode of no abode,
> Who sees all beings
> With the being of oneself
> And the being of oneself
> as that of all beings

From not holding to the other
As opposite from oneself
There is the essence of dharma[5]

One of the homework practices I often offer to students is to try and refrain from creating opposites for one week. If you're walking down the road, try not to categorize "short" as opposite from "tall," "black" as opposite from "white," "female" as opposite from "male," or "friend" as opposite from "enemy." By not defining things as opposite from other things, we begin to look closely at gradients and nuances and take ourselves out of the illusory role of objective witnesses somehow at a remove from contact with life. Instead we begin to participate in a reality where we don't set ourselves apart from the flux of what we are perceiving. Just like when, during our practice of deep yoga postures, we enter completely into the realm of clarity and feeling, or when we watch the breath until we dissolve into breathing itself, we refrain from making opposites only to find that the witness that so dominates our moment-to-moment perceptions dissolves and we become one with that of which we are aware. We become the other as we see how the origin and completion of nonviolent practices begin through clarity of attention in this moment, free from the need to make everything into oppositional categories that we believe to be real.

The term "dharma" that completes the passage above describes yoga teachings as a description of how things actually are. "Dharma" is not so much an anthropocentric truth but a natural law of the material world, observable, just as change is, in everything.

PSYCHOLOGY AND ETHICS

Psychology is the organization of experience. We cannot take in the world through any means other than our sense organs and the mind. In fact, the body and mind might be the largest part of the world we can ever know, simply by the fact that mind, body, and world are inseparable. You cannot read these words without eyes or think about this text without mind or feel the book you are holding without skin, bones, and physiology. We perceive body and mind via body and mind; and the sense organs organize sense data in a process we call psychology, which by definition is always psychosomatic.

Since we all organize our experience differently, especially since we all have sense organs and minds uniquely conditioned and habituated, it is important to remember that we cannot approach ethics without taking subjectivity into account. Subjectivity means that we are always dealing with our unique perceptual viewpoints determined by our bodies and minds, which are in turn conditioned by culture.

Taking this a step further, we may wonder if human subjectivity should be the primary measurement for ecological decision making. I cannot know what a fish feels when caught by a net or hook, nor can I know what my students feel as they sit with turbulent thoughts or emotions. Our decisions as human beings, because of our subjectivity, tend to revolve around what we need, or rather, what we think other living beings need.

Integrating ethics, psychology, and spirituality has a long but often forgotten history. To provide a basis for rethinking ethical action, we are using the *Yoga-Sūtra* attributed to Patañjali. Not only have I been studying and teaching this text for many years, I have been practicing the ethics and meditative techniques described in its short and dense volume, continually oscillating between ethics as a set of guidelines and ethics as a visceral expression of nonduality. In addition to teaching yoga postures, philosophy, meditation, and breathing practices, I am also a psychotherapist. One of the biggest differences between Western psychotherapy and Yoga teachings is that Yoga begins with ethics. In Western psychology we talk a great deal about professional ethics and how to speak with patients clearly and where the boundaries lie in our clinical work. But for a profession that perhaps more than any other profession helps people decide how to take action, therapists are not required to study, practice, or express their personal ethical guidelines. Perhaps ethics is one of the most neglected topics in our contemporary culture. I have tried to address this lacuna in a yearlong course designed for clinicians interested in integrating contemplative practice in their clinical work. Our focus is using ethics as a means for self-study. We meet together in small groups to check in about the way that our mental state affects our ethical choices throughout the week. Every week the participants speak with one another and describe actions that are skillful and actions that have been unskillful. This approach helps them integrate conversations about ethics in their work with their clients, because they see the way that motivation determines the kind of world we perceive.

I am also a father. Wearing the hats of householder, parent, teacher, therapist, and yoga practitioner provides me not only with a transdisciplinary perspective but also with a motivation to tie together these seemingly diverse perspectives in order to see their inherent union. Yoga is a householder practice. If yoga does not support the quality of our family relationships, the health of our community, the way we source and eat our food, the way we feel in mind and body, how is it beneficial? Ramana Maharishi described ethical action and union with the world as one and the same. He compares the yogi with a bucket in well: It is water with water all around.[6] Unfortunately, spiritual practices have a long history of being mixed up with political ideologies where the elites ratchet up the goals of practice in such a way that the householders feel they can't practice until after their family commitments are over. This leads to a split where the monastic and lay communities are told that their possibilities of awakening are not equal. This leaves many lay practitioners feeling that family life is not a valid form of yoga. Mothering, breast-feeding, laundry—these are valid forms of yoga practice because they are expressions of intimacy in action. Again, yoga is a householder practice.

Like love at first sight, the immediate feeling of reverence and to-getherness, even in the midst of parenting, brings about the will to take action. When we stop in a moment of fury and take a deep breath, that immediate and physical pause stops our reactive instinct and turns us not just inward but also forward toward a clear comprehension of what is occurring. The great historian and scholar of yoga Mircea Eliade, having served his spiritual apprenticeship in the holy city of Rishikesh, decided after his meditative experiences to replace the word "*ec*stacy" (*extase*) with "*in*stacy" (*entase*), because "ectasy" seemed too marked by exteriority. We are not trying to achieve something that is outside of us. Eliade felt that intacy better describes the way that sitting still and noticing what moves through awareness brings about an indwelling attention that does not just stop inside oneself but serves to connect us with the pulse of life. In other words we don't rely on the external; instead we turn inward only to find that the pause of turning inward leads us outward again but outward in a whole different sense. We find that through a process of stilling the elaborations of the mind, the external and internal become one and the same and all opposites come to an end.

Described either as a circle with internal spokes relating one part of the circle with another, or as a net in which every strand is intimately tied to every other, the way we perceive and take action ripples through all systems, creating a seamless and circular mandala. The family is a mandala, farmers and cities are spokes in the mandala, and community and water form the flow.

We study our mental states in order to settle them and finally move with grace and attunement. Moving beyond our likes and dislikes opens us up to the relational matrix of life. In fact we can define healthy relationship as the ability to take in someone or something without superimposing our biases and expectations on them.

THE BOTTOMLESS MIND

The meditative experiences articulated by Patañjali in the *Yoga-Sūtra*, and most especially his teachings on samādhi (integration) and svarupa shunya (emptiness of self-image), have made me realize that what passes for "normal" in today's mental-health vocabulary and criteria is a low-grade form of illness. I have come across this stance before, especially in the philosophical work of Michel Foucault, Deleuze and Guattari, R. D. Laing and many others, but sitting still and seeing the reactive and highly conditioned nature of my own busy mind and body made me realize that I've hardly been present much in my short time on earth. This is not an overstatement. Most of us are so caught up in the conceptual mind, juggling ideas, making plans, keeping things together, that we've never really looked into the nature of our own minds and bodies and most especially what it means to be a self or to have a self. Even our bodies are sleeping. We are living in an attention-deficit society caught between passive laxity on one hand and hyperactivity on the other. We need some technique so that we can reestablish attention in our daily lives and bring this attentiveness to bear on the important matters we all face personally and collectively.

We practice yoga postures to move deeply into the workings of the body, which are none other than the simple workings of the universe, and also to prepare the body not for something in the future but to take in what is occurring here and now.

When all of the fluctuations of the mind settle and the reactive patterning is suspended, one wakes up to samādhi, which is the end of the construction of a separate self, even momentarily. The word *samādhi* is not an esoteric or utopian dream, but rather a description of what it means to be so fully present that there is experience unfolding in which you are participating without separation. You are so fully in what you are doing that you disappear. It's not that you don't exist, but that when you are completely present you are not creating a separate "me." You will no doubt have had this kind of experience in your life; where you have been so fully engaged in present experience—making art, making love, meditation, conversation—that the sense of being a self dissolves. This is hard to describe in words. In meditative realization you begin to see that you don't practice to achieve enlightenment; instead, practice is simply a manifestation of enlightenment. Though the yamas may appear to be a path *to* samādhi, they are also a creative expression *of* samādhi.

BEYOND THE FAMILIAR

We can no longer live a spiritual life and pursue a path of awakening divorced from the stark realities of ecological disaster and personal alienation. In fact, these stark realities—personal, social, economic, and ecological duḥkha—give rise to spiritual practice in the first place. (*Duḥkha* is a Sanskrit term that can be translated as "suffering, discontent, lack, or unsatisfactoriness." Considered by both Yogic and Buddhist schools to be a characteristic of life, the psychological meaning of duḥkha is even though it may seem that suffering is something that comes from outside oneself—for example, from the government, or childhood, or one's body—suffering is actually self-generated.) When we see suffering, we want to know how to deal with it because in our heart of hearts we cannot bear continuous affliction. The economic systems we all share may always provide uneven distribution of security, but even so, there is a much deeper security that we all desire. The forests need security; the fish need security; the mind needs security. We all find ourselves bereft of answers in the face of the kind of limited means and ends we all face now with the convergence of species extinction, deforestation, poverty, climate change, and war. The primary life systems of this planet—its veins and arteries and lungs and waterways—are slowly shutting down. Our ethical traditions certainly know how to deal with one issue at a time, and we also have knowledge bases that can deal with suicide and homicide, but we as of now have no strong approach in dealing with biocide—the devastating and irreversible collapse of the major living systems of this planet.

This very body is the earth itself; the earth is our body. The *Shiva Samhita* describes this interplay of macrocosm and microcosm:

> Within this body exists Mount Meru, the seven continents, lakes, oceans, mountains, plains, and the protector of these plains . . . all the stars and planets, the sacred river crossings and pilgrimage centers . . . the whirl of the sun and the moon, which are the causes of creation and annihilation. Likewise it contains ether, air, fire, water and earth. He who knows all this is a yogi. There is no doubt about that.[7]

We usually use the term *ethics* to mean humans and their relationships to each other. This is called interhuman ethics. According to yoga, however, we see ethics as human beings in relationship in a more general sense, without determining relational limits. Thinking of relationship as one "thing" in relationship to another discrete "thing" is dualistic psychology based on binary perception and is exactly what yoga aims to see through.

When we say that everything is connected, we still see that from human eyes, don't we? How do we operate *as* the natural world?

One particle reveals another set of building blocks under which lie another set and another set, ad infinitum. Nowhere is there an inadequacy of relations. To think we are not always in relationship is only a mind in duḥkha. We are suffering from skewed vision. Can we announce that *yoga* is a political word as much as a spiritual one? Can we not say that yoga stands against division in all its manifestations, psychological, racial, and economic. Yoga is the fact and flesh of interconnectivity.

YOGA DESCRIBES THE inherent unity of all relations as a priori, and the splitting of the world into "me" and "that" as a secondary human action. In other words, before we fragment things into subject and object—a "me" and a world outside of me, or a mind inside a body inside a world—everything is already yoked as it is. One of the clearest descriptions of this attitude comes from the Polish poet Wisława Szymborska in her poem "View with a Grain of Sand":

> We call it a grain of sand,
> but it calls itself neither grain nor sand.
> It does just fine without a name,
> whether general, particular,
> permanent, passing, incorrect, or apt.
>
> Our glance, our touch mean nothing to it.
> It doesn't feel itself seen and touched.
> And that it fell on the windowsill
> is only our experience, not its.
> For it, it is no different from falling on anything else
> with no assurance that it has finished falling
> or that it is falling still.
>
> The window has a wonderful view of the lake,
> but the view doesn't see itself.
> It exists in this world
> colorless, shapeless,
> soundless, odorless, and painless.
>
> The lake's floor exists floorlessly,
> and its shore exists shorelessly.
> Its water feels itself neither wet nor dry
> and its waves to themselves are neither singular or plural.
> They splash deaf to their own noise
> on pebbles neither large nor small.
>
> And all this beneath a sky by nature skyless
> in which the sun sets without setting at all

and hides without hiding behind an unminding cloud.
The wind ruffles it, its only reason being
that it blows.

A second passes.
A second second.
A third.
But they're three seconds only for us.

Time has passed like a courier with urgent news.
But that's just our simile.
The character is invented, his haste is make-believe,
His news inhuman.[8]

If what moves through the sense organs is "inhuman," it is so because we haven't got hold of it yet. When data moves through the sense
organs, it gets sculpted, formed, and manipulated and changes from
mere "data" to "in-formation."

Our sense organs are organs of selection, never mind what we do
with experience when we attempt to categorize what has been received
and put it into words. The kind of action we take in relation to the
natural world, to each other, and to ourselves determines the kind of
world we perceive; the way we perceive in turn influences the way we
organize our experiences, our decisions to act, and ultimately the kind
of world we live in. Action and perception create an infinite feedback
loop we call karma. Social and ecological engagement, psychology, and
spiritual practice are not separate paths. At base, the yamas describe
responsiveness born of realization. From this perspective, social or ecological action is actually what and who you are.

A theme that emerges throughout yoga teachings and praxis is not
mastery over the body or language or the mind but rather a retuning
that returns us to the wild ecology that is our true home. This does not
mean that we need to leave cities and move into forests or claim some

piece of the earth as an absolute utopia. We need to reattune to the complex interdependence of the air and earth and mind and heart so that we can return to our animated ecological mind and reactivate this wisdom in contemporary times because *these are our times,* and without increased wisdom and attentiveness, they'll pass us by.

CHAPTER THREE

LACK

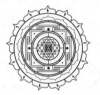

We live in complicated times. We seek, but we don't necessarily find, the ultimate things we long to experience—contentment, joy, love, inner peace. Our lives are too often overloaded with demands: that we should be successful, rich, beautiful and famous; but this just adds to our inner stress and turmoil. The media constantly bombard us with images reminding us of our "lack" . . . and we so often feel like failures.[1]

S INGER AND SOCIAL activist Annie Lennox strikes the heart of our incessant strivings: lack and our attempts to fill it. Not only do "the media constantly bombard us" with "lack," we find ourselves willing the lack only to feel its vacuum once again. "Lack" is an excellent translation of the Sanskrit term "duḥkha" because it describes the felt sense of being unsatisfied. Do you ever feel there is a gnawing sense that there is something you lack? How much of your life have you looked outward to try and fill this inadequacy? How much does this sense of emptiness or lack motivate your choices and ambitions?

Usually at the center of the personality, many of us feel and are motivated by a sense that something is missing. Sometimes even as we approach deep stillness, before the mind and body settle into calmness, we first experience fear, distraction, and a hint that something inside of us is missing, incomplete, ill at ease, or even threatenening. The sense of self has a shadow that informs its basic structure and, by extension, influences our actions and core values. Lack is the shadow of self-image. We cling to self in order to maintain the illusion that the shadow is not there, and the more we run away from the feelings of incompleteness that arise as we begin to settle into stillness, the further we entrench this shadow and its corresponding feelings deficiency. Our sense of self is a construct, an ever-changing process, which doesn't have any ontological reality of its own (re-representing ourselves to ourselves).

Because self-representation lacks any reality of its own, any stable ground, the sense of self is haunted by what David Loy, in his groundbreaking book *Lack and Transcendence*, calls a sense of lack. By translating duḥkha as lack, Loy returns the term to its existential base, or rather lack of base, in the center of the personality. The origin of this sense of lack is our inability to open up to the emptiness, and boundlessness, of the self. While the negative aspect of feeling lack is the drive to fill this emptiness with egoistic ambitions like romantic love or the accumulation of money, the positive aspect of lack is that recognizing the inherent insubstantiality of the self expands our experience of who and what we are and connects us to the ecology of being alive. The self cannot be grounded with anything outside itself because, as a fiction, it never existed in the first place. Insofar as we're unable to cope with that emptiness, insofar as we deny it and shy away from it, we experience it as a sense of shortcoming.

The interesting thing about the external forms of gratification that we use to fill this lack at our core is that when they disappear or decay (like the loss of a lover, job, money, or status), they return us to the basic truth that nothing outside of ourselves can ultimately create a solid ground out of which we can find peace. The body is always grounded, but it is grounded in a way that self-constructed images of ourselves never can be. "Freedom from wanting," Patañjali states, "unlocks the real purpose of existence."[2]

As a shadow, lack refers to the fact that no "thing" has any inherent "thingness," because "it" lacks an ongoing substantiative core. For example, if I look at where the wall and ceiling meet, especially if I get up really close, I can't actually find the border of the wall. The wall in this room is blue and the ceiling white, yet if I took a microscope, there would be no clean line dividing blue and white in a linear way. If I can't find the distinction between wall and ceiling, it's not because there is no wall; it's just because "wall" and "ceiling" are designations. To push this further, there can be no ceiling without a wall, and I would not be able to name "ceiling" unless it is in relation to a wall.

This is an easy line of thinking with regard to objects. But whenever there is an object, there is also a subject. How can we find the place where subject ends and object begins? Where does my ear end and sound begin? Where do these words end and the mind begin? When I breathe, how far into the nostrils or respiratory system does the breath have to flow before it's part of my body? If I eat a piece of bread, at what point is it no longer bread and now a part of me? At what point do the rivers meet in this very body? Where do thoughts begin and end in the mind? Where does the water that makes up the majority of this human body meet up with the great waters of the rivers, lakes, and oceans?

Even if I look into my eyes in the reflection of a mirror, I can't find the source or essence of "Michael." Supposing the eyes are windows of the soul, revealing what is most "me," no matter how deep I look into the retina, pupil, or dilating movements and shifts of the eyeball in all its colorful array, all I can find is temporary patterns and color and shape; I cannot find any "Michael" in this process. Michael seems to be an "object" that the mind has created and superimposed on the shifting form of the eye. The sum of the parts to which I give the name "eye" reveals no self at all. In fact, with sustained attentiveness, I can't find any part of the eye that I can relate to as me or mine.

IMPERMANENCE, SELF, AND LACK

In terms of how this impacts our daily life, we come to see that if a subject only occurs in relation to an object, every time we turn people, things, feelings, or thoughts into objects, we build a sense of self that is split off from the world. The root of all misconception stems from the false apprehension of things as objects outside of "me." The root affliction we all face is being caught up in emotions and states of mind that we believe to be real, which gives us a sense of *being* real, when in fact, all states of mind are conditioned phenomena arising and passing away.

We all have times when we feel something we'd rather not, and instead of opening up to it, we avoid it and tell ourselves stories about what we are feeling rather than actually feeling the arising emotion. Sometimes, for example, we have so many ideas about what we are feeling that we don't allow the feelings to arise and move on naturally, and instead, we fix the feeling in time and space by associating to it, thereby turning the feeling into an object for the mind. When we create an object out of the feeling, we give it substantiality; we give it a separate self. This serves to keep the mind distracted from the ephemeral nature of the feeling, and instead of letting it pass on, we get entangled in thoughts about what we are feeling rather than dropping into the arising feeling itself, which, when felt, will pass on and give way to something else. All we have to do is gently touch the feeling and observe how it comes and goes, and in doing so, we touch the mind of no time, the body of no time, the feeling that is not governed by any thoughts or concepts. The mind that is no longer obsessed with time and how long something will last is the patient and bottomless mind we call pure awareness and that Patañjali names *puruṣa*. Even when we feel difficult feelings, pure awareness is hovering in the background, not as an actual thing or god or divine sense but as the plain and real truth that what we are experiencing is everything. The true way of practice is opened when we look deeply at these moments where time stops, the separation of self and object collapses, and wanting in all its forms comes to an end.

When we see that everything perceptible is arising and passing away, even in our own minds and bodies, we learn how to restrain from harmful conduct of body, speech, and mind, and contribute peace and centeredness to any situation, rather than compulsion or fury. Though states of anger, envy, jealousy, or greed have a strong and relentless purchase on us when we are caught up in them, they might also give way to entirely different states of mind just minutes later.

Everything is empty of its own being, or self-being, especially seen at a distance. If we try and find the center of a waterfall or a leaf, it's hard to discover. But the most problematical emptiness and lack for us has to do with our own sense of self. Our ideas about ourselves tend to generate grooves in the mind-body process that interrupt a natural inclination toward consideration of others and gloss over the truth of change. Our contraction around who we think we are obscures the fact that, at bottom, the self is intimately tied with everything before we split the world up into bits and pieces. Such splitting creates the sense of lack that then motivates us to find intimacy outside of us rather than loosening the self-created grip that holds us apart from the world.

We can tie in this truth of insubstantiality to the teachings of duḥkha. Although duḥkha is often translated into English as "suffering," when you look at the core teachings, duḥkha is obviously a much broader term that includes more general dissatisfaction, a basic frustration in our lives that we are never quite able to resolve. And this broader meaning of duḥkha includes a basic dissatisfaction connected to the conditioned nature of the self, which is always trying to find any way possible to ground itself. But if the self is just a construct, a story, an ongoing narrative, how can it ever feel truly grounded? There is a profound link between our basic dissatisfaction and our deluded sense of self, partly because the ego is always trying to become *something* even though such an ideal refers to a perfection impossible to achieve. This is where Western psychology leaves off.

From a relational, psychological, and existential point of view, we're worried about the future death of some self we think exists, but in essence there is something deeper operating; namely, we're frightened about the fact that, right now, we don't exist in the first place. We come to see that letting go of the egoistic constructions does not take us to a new personality with a new kind of self, but rather exposes the fact that a self does not exist in the first place, because it is a mirage, an image, an illusion.

Duḥkha is not due to an impermanence that is going to occur to the body one day in the future in the form of death. It is the coming together and coming apart of the personality from moment to moment. This is no metaphor. There is no solid and continuing "me." The self is groundless.

It takes several generations for monarch butterflies to complete their annual migration. The flight patterns are maintained even though the individuals are constantly changing. This analogy reminds us how we construct and reconstruct our memories, ideas, thoughts, and personalities, yet still maintain a persistent self. The body's cells are constantly turning over, yet we still continue to be recognizable to ourselves and others. Psychologically we have a self-image that seems to continue through this regeneration process, but ontologically there is no ongoing self below the images and ideas we have of it.

Anything that we repress, David Loy explains, is something that we're unwilling or unable to cope with, so we turn our attention away from it and continually look for outer forms of gratification. But if it's something really pressing—like sexuality for Freud—then it's not so easy for us to escape these always-occurring energies. Whether it's sexual energy, greed, or anger, all potential states of mind and body are going to find a way to return to awareness, which is what Freud called the "return of the repressed."[3] Freud coined the phrase "return of the repressed" to explain the existence of neurotic symptoms. He theorized that an unconscious thought or feeling would constantly press for access to the conscious mind in order to be discharged, to achieve balance, to come out into the light. The ego would be on constant alert to prevent the direct expression of the forbidden idea, but the idea would find a disguise and surface as a symptom. This also happens on a collective level. If we are not able to accept, acknowledge, and live with the experience of our own emptiness, then it will return as the various compulsive ways that we try to ground ourselves in the world, to make ourselves feel more real. But we can't ground ourselves externally.

Seeking pleasure through external means is a general preoccupation for almost all of us, but the particular form that it takes depends upon the kind of person you are and the kind of cultural context that you find yourself within. In the modern North American context, accumulating money is the culture's most significant "security project."[4] Collectively, we seem to believe that more money will make us more real and feel increasingly complete. But there are also other basic security projects, especially fame and the forms of sexual desire that often masquerade as romantic completion. These are three of the common ways we try to overcome our sense of inadequacy and ground ourselves in the world, except "the world" in this case is a human-centered world created out of fear and an exaggerated belief that money, romantic love, or notoriety will give us solid grounding and existential rootedness.

Turning to spiritual practice is the way that humans have tried to understand and resolve their sense of lack.[5] In a way, all religions are systems that have tried to deal with the self's sense of paucity.

Like any symptom, lack is both a cause and symptom of discontent. Inadequacy is only the negative aspect of something that's much greater—something that is, in fact, potentially transformative. Lack also has a positive side. To summarize, it's our ungroundedness—a kind of bottomless hole at the very core of our being—that we usually experience as a shortcoming, because there is no way to ground the personality in something outward. How can you ground something that is only a moment-by-moment construction and without a solid core? Because we're so uncomfortable with or even terrified of this ungroundedness, we experience it as a sense of inferiority that we flee from. But if we can open up to that ungroundedness at our core, if we can let go and yield to it, then we find that it's the source of our creativity and our spirituality; that at the very core of our being there's something else there, something formless that cannot be grasped, something that transcends the self and yet is the basis of the self.

MONEY = ENERGY

We feel lack most acutely as we try and fill it. If we want more money, as an example, it's hard to bring awareness to the nature of wanting; it is much easier to focus on the object itself. We tell ourselves we don't need more, or perhaps we are satisfied and we intellectualize away the desire. But within the feeling of wanting, there is an important knot to untie. Is it possible to feel the want without focusing on the object—whether the object is money or another person or one's own body? If I crave money, can I learn how to work with the craving so that whatever form the object takes becomes insignificant? Instead, the state of wanting (*rāga*) is what's focused on, not the object.

Psychoanalyst Adam Phillips writes:

> What are we wanting when we want money? And that means not only, of course, when we want more money, but also when we want less. Is there a part of ourselves for which money is not, indeed never can be, the currency? And is this part of ourselves, however described, progressively silenced in a culture that speaks in money, and is therefore progressively driven to distraction?[6]

Money can never be a satisfying object because money is only a symbolic exchange. Even when we save money and accumulate enormous retirement estates, and even if we never dip into our accounts, it is still something we imagine will offer security in the future. Even when we are not actively "doing something" with our money, at a psychological level we can't help using the money for symbolic purpose. Money, at a symbolic level, describes what we most want and most fear and is instrumental in reinforcing individual and collective patterns of lack and compulsion.

Sometimes the symbol of money becomes so physical we enter numb states while shopping. "I can't feel anything," someone said to me recently in an attempt to describe her addiction to shopping. "It's like an out-of-body experience. When I'm tired or bored or sad or have nothing to do, it gives me something to do."

From another perspective we might ask, In what ways does shopping serve to reinforce boredom or loneliness? As she described her experience, she went on to say, "It's like you and I talking right now. If I have to look you in the eye, I'm scared of what that will feel like. Even so, I don't know what I want."

"Well what do you want?" I ask her quietly.

"The funny thing is what I want most is to look you in the eye. What I want most is to stop shopping. What I want most is just to stop all this distraction. That's why I'm practicing. But now I'm realizing that what I really want when I'm shopping is just this feeling of looking into someone's eyes."

When we try and ground ourselves through shopping and distraction, we are actually trying to connect with a deeper sense of who we are and our place in the world. But we are moving in the wrong direction. Intimacy arrives when renunciation occurs, not through accumulation and the duress of obsessive fixation, but through participating in what is happening here and now.

RENUNCIATION AND INTIMACY

Who is telling myself the story of myself? On what basis do I feel the need to fill up this lack? Am I creating the story of "self" from moment to moment or does the momentum of the narrative keep the story going?

Our ideas about ourselves are tested in the world and in various so-cial interactions. These interactions, in turn, provide a basis for crystal-lizing and refining our identity and who we want or believe ourselves to be. This social mirroring gives us a sense of ourselves that is constantly changing through different relationships but lacks, at bottom, a sub-stantial core that is unchanging. The role that others play in our cre-ation and experience of ourselves is never ending; there can be no final completion. Yet the self is not simply a social construction, as many psychologists suggest, because even the social aspects of being human rely in every way on the body, which in turn relies on the earth and all its complexity and life. While we humans are certainly cultural fig-ures, we are also biological and organic. The human mind and body are formed in a living landscape, and yoga teachings from ethics to medita-tion, postures to breathing practices are an attempt to reorient us to this landscape and the natural function of awareness. What if we imagine awareness to be the natural ecology of mind?

When we feel a sense of insufficiency we tend to turn outward to find value reflected back to us. While this is important in the early stages of development, turning outward becomes an inappropriate direction when we begin searching for the nature of the mind itself. No mental ego can ever achieve a perfectly grounded state, because it's made up of constantly changing interactions. By seeking recognition in people and things, the ego is always trying to ground itself, creating a tension that jeopardizes its importance and leaves room for existential inquiry to arise.

If the sense of lack is always present, perhaps it is something that does not need to be filled? Whenever we feed the lack with external objects, the lack actually increases. The mind emerges from processes intimately bound with other processes, not from static substance. We subsist within this ongoing flux as an ongoing flux.

This table describes the characteristics of duḥkha in the form of per-vasive lack:

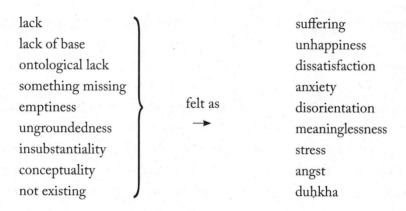

lack			suffering
lack of base			unhappiness
ontological lack			dissatisfaction
something missing			anxiety
emptiness	felt as	disorientation
ungroundedness	→	meaninglessness
insubstantiality			stress
conceptuality			angst
not existing			duḥkha

HEALING LACK

The opposite of lack is openness and intimacy. The opposite of duḥkha is serenity and karuṇā, compassion. Compassion is being with the reality of lack without seeing lack as something that needs to be filled. When we no longer treat lack as a vacuum, compassion arises through intimacy because instead of self-image being something we need to fortify (which only serves to increase the lack), we let go and find ourselves flourishing in this vast, shifting, and interconnected life.

To discover the fact that there is no substantial self to fill or to become is to touch the heart of this practice. In fact, this is what practice aims toward. The patterns of relations beneath craving and habitual wanting create the ground upon which we live, and that ground is *this* ground. Such an insight is an invaluable and indispensible guide.

Relational life can never be framed in a book on yoga or in a series of rules to follow. Relationship *is* daily life. When I refine my sensitivity to myself and others, when I take my time chewing, listening to others with more patience, becoming clearer in my speech, I am living a life tuned in to the web, and the self is not my first concern. By being more myself, I feel affinity with all of life, not just the preferred parts of existence that I tune in to when I need the world to be something *for* me. There is a seed of egoism in all of us. But there is also the desire to wake up and be free of narrow versions of ourselves. It's exactly the same with suffering and happiness. If we have not moved fully through the realms of suffering, our happiness will be incomplete. Suffering is the foundation for happiness, anxiety the beginning of change. I discover that there "has never been any lack, because there has never been any self-existing self apart from the world."[7] This discovery is the heart of yoga, namely, dropping away the subjectively governed consciousness.

Until we see the relationship between filling our sense of lack and the ways we get entangled in our endless egotistic desires, it is difficult to be tuned in to the birdsong and the rivers, to our lovers and our friends. From difficulty, we are moved to listen. The unconscious actions we've taken have created disastrous effects in the ecological, psychological, and economic spheres. The cycles of life and death and the complexities in the web of life are movements much greater than our individual human activity in one lifetime. Against this cosmic background, the span of a human life, the growth of a white pine, the experience of a jackrabbit are only brief movements in a cycle of ongoing change. Rachel Carson, author of the now famous classic from 1962, *Silent Spring*, describes relational attunement and the motivation for action in crystal clear words: "I could never again listen happily to a thrush song if I had not done all I could."[8]

CHAPTER FOUR

KARMA: CAUSALITY

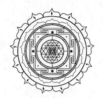

K ARMA IS THE law of cause and effect. Whenever we take an action, there is a corresponding though incalculable effect. In Indian philosophy, karma is considered a causal natural law in the same way we could say that gravity is a natural law of physics. Karma is not operated by some higher power or god that chooses what kind of effects will happen based on your actions in this or previous lifetimes; karma is not like some kind of Santa Claus that adds up your rights and wrongs and determines the feedback loop most appropriate for you.

Simply put, karma is the relationship between actions and their effects. Good actions tend to have positive effects, and actions with negative intention, like the desire to cause harm, have negative effects. Sometimes the effects are not immediate, like the relationship between parents and children, and at other times we can see immediately the hurt we cause in poor speech or the joy we create when we act out of genuine kindness.

In popular culture, the term karma is most often translated as "fate." The Sanskrit word "vipaka" refers more to fate, or the exclusive effect of previous actions, but karma differs from vipaka in that it describes the causal relationship between volitional action and the effect of that action. It's easiest to consider karma as a seed that is planted and then ripens. Sooner or later our actions, like seeds, will bear fruit.

Karma is not a way of pointing out a divine order or some kind of omnipotent creator god that keeps an eye on all that we do. Karma is also not some evolved superego that controls all aspects of our conscience. On one end of the spectrum we could believe that karma points out our predetermined destiny, a road map already created, whereby we simply "get what we deserve." On the other end of an exaggerated spectrum we find karma as pure luck, a random distribution of events and synchronicities all relative to one another. A grounded and practical understanding of karma is a middle path between the two extremes of free will and pure fate.

We want desperately, as humans caught up in a fleeting and imperfect world, to make sense and meaning of not only our personal lives but of life in general. It can be seductive to use karma to explain what is often unexplainable by using it as a metaphysical tool. Some people blame the tsunami of December 2004 on the karma of those affected by it. Others blamed Hurricane Katrina and the New Orleans flood in August 2005 on the karma of an American culture at war. While sometimes using karma in this way has great explanatory power, this logic is built on sand because the conditions that give rise to any one event are so complex that they are beyond reductionistic comprehension. Although there are some Indian uses of the term *karma* where it is weighted with metaphysical or existential fate, the yogi's notion of karma is equally balanced between actions and their effects, like multiple feedback loops, with the present moment being shaped both by past and by present actions; present actions shape not only the future but also the present. Furthermore, present actions need not be determined by past actions. In other words, there is always free will, although its range is somewhat dictated by the past.

We could say that the yamas on nonharming, honesty, nonstealing, wise use of energy, and nonacquisitiveness are based on the law of karma. Karma, in the context of the yamas, is a tool designed to help us see the intimate nature of all relationship. How I talk with you affects the quality of our communication, affecting how I feel, how you feel, and how others who come into contact with us feel about our contact in that moment. Karma is not some kind of spiritual air-mile system with merit and demerit added by some divine teller. Rather, karma points out the importance of purifying our actions of body, speech, and mind, so that the way we live our life benefits all with whom we are in relationship.

Often on retreat or in long courses, one of the group exercises we practice begins by reflecting on some of the ways we've acted unkindly over the day. In partnerships or in small groups we can notice where greed or anger, competitiveness or dishonesty took hold of us and influenced how we spoke or acted. Each person meets with the same partner every day for the duration of the course and describes where some action was taken that may have caused unwanted harm to another or even oneself, however slight. People meet their partner daily or weekly and simply note the way that actions of body, speech, or mind were unskillful. While at first this may seem like a very simple exercise, it challenges the group to bring awareness to every aspect of their day, raising attention to a level where we can study our actions, intentions, and the effect of our actions. The other person just listens, and then we switch. As we listen, we pass no judgment; we simply create an atmosphere in which our partner feels safe and encouraged to the degree that honesty feels natural. This is one of the ways we teach about causality. The kind of attention and steadiness we bring to our āsana practice now carries forth through the domain of speech and attentive listening, rolling the practice off the sticky mat and into the tangled world of communication. This is how we see the practice through.

What's important about exercises like these is that there is no determination of right or wrong action. This helps us open to the yamas as guidelines rather than universal absolutes based on idealized notions of perfection or purity. Karma in the context of the yamas becomes a lens through which we can see how the world hangs together, how things feed and rebound off one another. Seeing actions of body, speech, and mind in terms of causality challenges us to wake up and become more

sensitive and clear, flexible, and honest. When we practice honesty (satya) and ground our actions in nonviolence, we plant those very seeds as
future potentials. This is how we plant the seeds of culture. What kind
of seeds shall we plant?

THE IDIOM OF INTIMACY

Investigating the relationship between our intentions, actions, and the
effect of our actions, we literally transform our world. Most of, if not all
of, our global strife, comes down to the separation of humans from the
earth, from each other, and ultimately, from ourselves. This gives rise
to discontent and its corresponding symptoms: greed, anger, ignorance,
envy, anxiety, clinging, and distress. If yoga begins with relationship, the
cure for the world's symptoms of stress and dissatisfaction comes down
to a matter of perception. When we are acting in our own self-interest,
when competitiveness and greed, or anger and ill will, rule our minds
from moment to moment, we don't experience the world relationally;
we experience "it" as divided. Spiritual practice in everyday life manifests in any moment that the gap between form and formlessness dissolves. Every time you step into that gap, you step into enlightenment.[1]

Examine how your intentions deeply affect your mood and mode of
seeing. In meditative practice, when we are caught up in delusive thinking or cascading distraction, it's helpful to notice the attitude we bring
to the object we are noticing. Are we trying to get rid of a mental state
or emotion, or can we notice it and feel it clearly? Do we think a thorny
feeling in the body is permanent, or can we watch it change? Attitude
needs to be adjusted accordingly, and over time we begin to see the way
intention influences the quality of our awareness in any given moment.

If there is a world "out there," there must be a "me" in here; when
there is an object, there is a self. The more I treat the world of earth,
elements, and people as out there and separate from "me," the more
alienated I feel. In that alienation I can't see the nature of reality clearly

because I'm trapped in the world of things, just as I'm enclosed by the television of my mind with its constant stream of ideas and images. When I treat the world as an object, I become a solidified subject. I do this to myself. In relational terms, we become like ice cubes bouncing off one another in a cold pitcher of water. We race to work and step over each other, or we work in competition with one another. The simple truth is that rushing has become a habit for many of us and it has a negative effect on our mental, spiritual, and physical health. Watching the rush-hour race, I'm always amazed at how humans push and fight for their imagined right to be first. Even bicycling our son to his downtown school each morning, I find it hard not becoming aggressive in such polluted and congested traffic lanes. But if every action creates the universe, certainly another attitude is possible. Resentment and anger grow when there is separation, because separation entails alienation. Alienation, in turn, feeds aggression, conceit, and entitlement. The more I feel separated, the more cut off I am from knowing what your experience is. Without openness to the other, I turn the other into an object.

INTEGRAL PARTS OF AN INTEGRATED WHOLE

We are integral parts of this marvel we call life. What it means to be human has roots deeper than we may realize on the surface. All of life's roots are entangled. Even this evening, stepping out of a rural retreat cabin and looking up into the milky sky of northern stars, it takes time for the eyes, breath, and body to become receptive and quiet, especially after hours of writing and reading. When seduced by too much surface thinking and reactive states of mind, the interconnectivity we call life is obscured.

After teaching about karma, Patañjali offers the yoga practitioner an eight-limbed path of practice called Aṣṭāṅga Yoga, which is described as more like a web or a spoked hub than a linear format for practice,

because each limb connects intimately with every other limb. We can
think of the eight limbs as linear, with one stage leading to the next
like so:

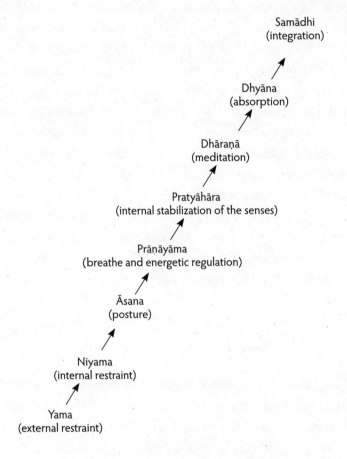

Fig. 1. Linear conception of the eight-limbed path.

The problem with this model of practice is that it creates the notion
that practice leads in a linear direction. Furthermore, it ratchets up the
practice of samādhi, making it seem especially holy or sacred when in
fact it only serves to clarify the other limbs through a constant retuning

quality of the attention span. Perhaps it's more accurate and healthy to
think of the eight limbs as circular:

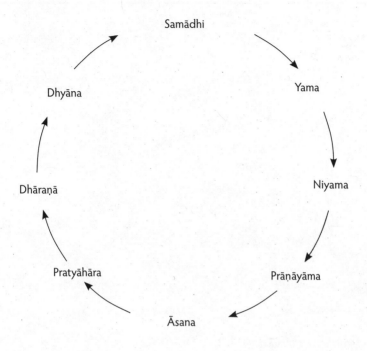

Fig. 2. Circular conception of the eight-limbed path.

What is helpful about the circular form is that we begin to see how
one stage may provide the ground for the next but also that samādhi—
waking up to the inherent integration of all things—is expressed
through our actions of the yamas. The yamas, in this model, become
expressions of samādhi.

However, we can reconceptualize the path by creating a concentric
image of practice that allows room for development, transformation,
and the refinement of unskillful habit energies. The concentric model
looks like this:

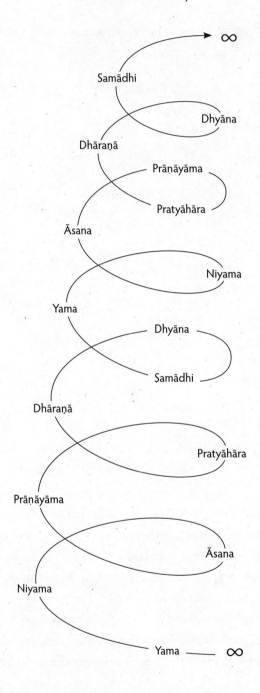

Fig. 3. Concentric conception of the eight-limbed path.

The concentric model of the eight limbs makes the yamas flow together as a supporting structure through which we move over and again, albeit with more and more stability. In this way the yamas are not simply sequential (as seen below). Instead, the yamas are samādhi put into action. This can be best understood as follows.

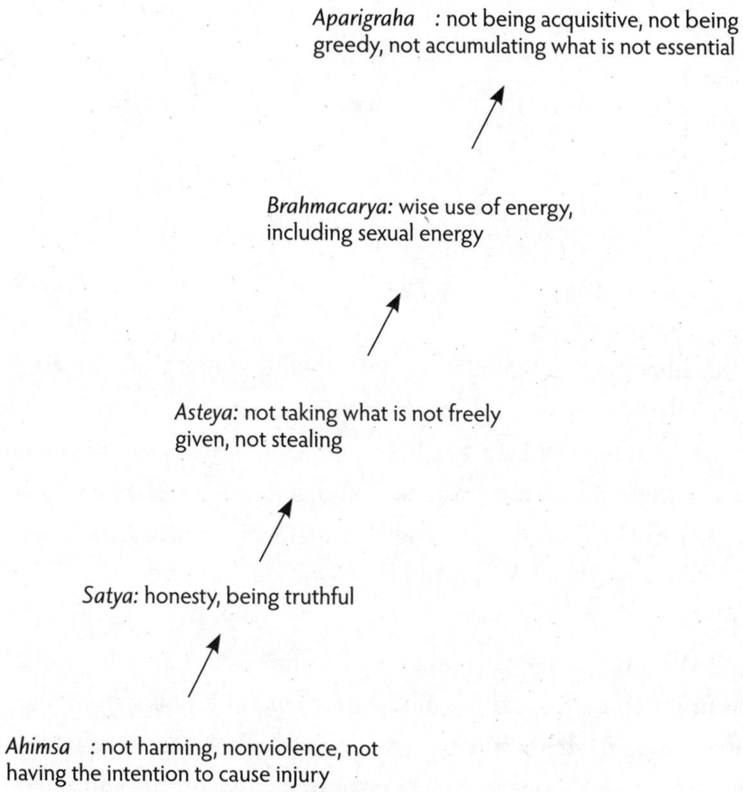

Aparigraha : not being acquisitive, not being greedy, not accumulating what is not essential

Brahmacarya: wise use of energy, including sexual energy

Asteya: not taking what is not freely given, not stealing

Satya: honesty, being truthful

Ahimsa : not harming, nonviolence, not having the intention to cause injury

Fig. 4. Linear conception of ethics.

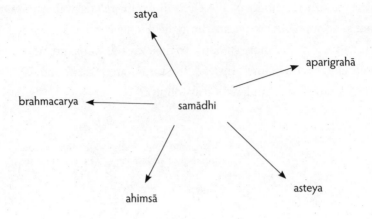

Fig. 5. Ethics as an expression of samādhi.

The liberating potential of karma in the context of the diagram above is that we see the way in which our actions are, at bottom, expressions of the integral whole. Secondly, our actions are always rising up in response to particular circumstances so that karma is seen to be creative potential rather than the ancient Brahmanic notion of karma as fate. Here is how one teacher puts it:

> Who you are—what you come from—is not anywhere near as important as the mind's motives for what it is doing right now. Even though the past may account for many of the inequalities we see in life, our measure as human beings is not the hand we've been dealt, for that hand can change at any moment. We take our own measure by how well we play the hand we've got. If you're suffering, you try not to continue the unskillful mental habits that would keep that particular karmic feedback going. If you see that other people are suffering, and you're in a position to help, you focus not on their karmic past but your karmic opportunity in the present: Someday you may find yourself in the same pre-

dicament that they're in now, so here's your opportunity to act in the way you'd like them to act toward you when that day comes.[2]

Ecology, psychology, and spirituality are sciences of context. They return our tendency toward self-interest to the wider and deeper ground of relationship. This is how we cultivate wisdom and compassion, the chief concerns of any spiritual path. "When the[se] components are practiced," Patañjali comments in the second chapter of his *Yoga-Sūtra*, "impurities dwindle; then, the light of understanding can shine forth, illuminating the way to discriminative awareness."[3] The yamas turn our practice toward relational life and in doing so, clarify the ingredients that contribute to the choices we make, because there is an echo in everything we do. It's the clarity of the mind, Patañjali suggests, that leads to viveka, creative and discriminating awareness.

Patañjali is a realist, not an idealist. We are not in search of a set of rules to follow, nor is yoga practice a practice of dogma. Realization of and commitment to interconnection and interdependence forms the overarching ethical code for the practicing yogin. The yamas are strategies for learning how to take action, though the yamas do not prescribe what specific action one should take in a specific situation: That is up to each of us.

A CULTURE OF CONSUMPTION OR CONNECTION?

Causality reminds us that every cause has an effect and every effect becomes the cause of future actions. Psychological change, then, is inseparable from spiritual awakening. If there is nowhere to go, what is *here* becomes valuable and worth tending.

There is an assumption in the way we talk about actions and the effects of our actions that there is some kind of natural law that will take care of everyone. Perhaps that natural law is science, or economics, or government policy, or, at a more psychological level, the belief that our conscience will get the better of us if our activities are exploitative to others or ourselves. Unfortunately, none of these assumptions have proved correct. Human actions and economic policies have, over the last several centuries, been determined by calculations of cost and expense, profit and loss, risk and benefit, which all aim to "optimize" the means that pertain to a specific end: growth and profit. But a real response to the reality of inequality must also come from the heart, not the two-column accounting system; otherwise we just keep bumping into ourselves.

In the two-column accounting system, designed to account for income and expense, there is little room for a column that measures accountability, social responsibility, ecological effect, and so on. Thus, it does not account for real costs. Additional (and invisible) columns are usually the responsibility of study groups or policymakers whose perspective is not built fundamentally, even operationally, into the two-column accounting system. Don't we need to take far more into account? If body and mind *are* endless, aren't the permutations and combinations also endless?

Karma teaches us that the first measure of accounting for our actions is in terms of consequences. Since we are always discovering new ends and means to consume and produce, we need to continually look at the consequences of our actions. Unrestrained materialism and ecological integrity exist in an absolute contradiction. We cannot continue to consume and produce at the velocity we are now. The result is a steady erosion of our well-being and the earth's delicate and complex balance. The root of the degradation is the endlessly invasive and expansive force of capital, gnawing away at the threads of ecological integrity and exceeding, with its inexorable pressure to expand, the earth's capacity to deal with ecological destabilization. We are greedy, and to deal with our sense of lack and disconnectedness, we pursue the accumulation of capital to try and ground us. We seek retirement security and other forms of financial safety in order to make us feel grounded. But where does it end?

Tending to relationship as another facet of practice synchronizes the mind and body with the heart of others, guaranteeing a natural rhythm to our lives based on nonseparation and tolerance, thus guaranteeing an internal sense of authenticity, credibility, and purpose. As we breathe in and breathe out, we are in constant and changing relational existence. Let us not squander our resources and creative capacities in distraction and aversion—we can certainly wake up with more heartfelt and creative responses to our global and personal ills and reverse the tide of frenzied self-destruction. Morality is an expression of your true nature and how it functions with the world. Do not drift through your life!

In stillness we can reconfigure our intentions and return to what is life-affirming. The yamas are not some final arbiter of right and wrong—we all are. In *Civil Disobedience,* Thoreau reminds us that even if one person withdraws his or her support from an unjust government or culture, it begins a cycle that will reverberate and grow.[4] An ethics governed by karma is an expression of the truth of interconnectedness and a compelling guideline for conduct in the world. Morality is not girded to social structures—it's an embodied expression of your basic wisdom, your basic nature, your whole body, breath, and mind. There is a kinship built into everything, and our realization of this is encapsulated by the term "yoga."

CHAPTER FIVE

AHIMSĀ:
NONVIOLENCE

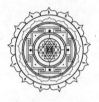

The covetous man is ever in want.

—HORACE, *Epistles*

It is blasphemy to say that nonviolence can be
practiced by individuals and never by nations, which
are composed of individuals.

—M. K. GANDHI

I N SEEKING ALTERNATIVES to violence in a case of conflict, there
is never just one alternative to a problem. Nonviolence seeks to clear
the mind of the delusion of rightness. You must have convictions, and
you must act on those convictions even though new evidence may cause
you to change your mind the next day. You have to act on the convictions you have today, or you will never act at all. But there is a difference
between a conditioned conviction and a view that is clung to.

The veneer of culture is often very thin, and while there is good in
every person, human beings are not innately nonviolent. Or maybe we

are? In either case, nonviolence can be taught and it can be learned, thereby taking the next great step in human evolution to the place where humans can take in multiple perspectives and become more flexible, tolerant, patient, and motivated to act for the welfare of ecology as a whole. Ecological awareness begins in one's own body and extends through community in all directions. Community grows deep roots when we help each other thrive. As Annie Dillard reminds us, "we live in all we seek"—there is no separation to begin with.[1] Everything I encounter supports, sustains, and creates me.

However, when we devise cultural strategies like war and social or ecological exploitation, we paradoxically feel more real because we secure ourselves by projecting our lack onto others. Isn't it strange how domination gives us the temporary illusion that we are right and real? When we create an object, we feel more like a self, and when a country creates an enemy, it reinforces the self-identity we call nationalism. War, as an example, secures our sense of self because the more we invest in creating enemies, the more we understand our place in the world and thus feel some sense of security even though such security is fleeting and inconsistent. Such exploitation is the opposite of renunciation: no synchronization, no intimacy, no togetherness.

This morning's newspaper headlines have begun to look like the headlines of every morning paper:

- AIDS Death Toll in Africa May Reach 100 Million by 2025
- Indonesian Quake Leaves 4,300 Dead and 200,000 Homeless
- U.N. Urges U.S. to Shut Guantanamo Prison
- West's Failure over Climate Change "Will Kill 182 Million Africans"
- U.N.'s Annan Wants U.S., Europe to Consider Force in Darfur
- 100 Days On, Pakistan Quake Survivors under Constant Threat
- China and India Hold Key to World's Riches or Ruin—Report
- Groups Demand Treaty to Ban International Gun Trade

Underneath these statistics we find ecological, economic, and social distress, but we also see interconnectedness. The practice of yoga is a practice of being with the reality of what is. Arriving in the present moment is sometimes painful because we stop and see our past choices and the unconsciousness in many of our activities. When we see the shadow of our actions, we can get motivated to change our habits.

Nonviolence is the essence of such change. This takes courage and lots of hard work. The momentum of habit sometimes seems unstoppable. Although "civilization," as a word, is taken to embrace the rise of cities, the elements of a civilized nature include the ability for humans to live in large clusters together. And these qualities include the development of an individualism that also accommodates the diversity of others, an individualism that is the opposite of tribalism and fanaticism. The industrialized West has not yet shown the qualities of a civilized nature, only the achievements of industrialism and competition. When integrated with our modern needs and ways of life, the nonaggressive roots of yoga offer us a multifaceted and resilient ethical way of life.

Industrialism is such an all-consuming impulse that it's hard to think outside the box. In fact we have interiorized the aspects of industrial materialism to the extent that we treat our own bodies as resources that should keep up with the impossible pace of increased productivity. The body, however, just can't keep up. We tend to forget that *we*—our bodies—are nature. The way we control and repress our own bodies and feelings is reflected in our treatment of all other life.

Despair is not a helpful mode of action. When I read these headlines, I imagine that this is what it feels like when a child loses his or her home. The world we are growing with is being radically changed in very upsetting ways. Nihilism and despair are not helpful responses because our attitude penetrates everything we do and negativity only serves to reinforce apathy and anger. Ninety-five percent of all the species that we've ever documented have disappeared. Evolution is taking a curious course, but at the same time, we have no idea what that course is going to be. It's our job to bear witness and take appropriate action, and how that action comes to fruition is a matter of personal expression.

Notions of a spiritual practice in which "I" can be saved but the other forms of creation cannot is simply untenable through the lens of samādhi. If there is ecological intimacy throughout this biosphere, then we are all in this movement together. When I have the tools to work with my capacity for apathy, distraction, laxity of attention, or even hyperactivity, I have more clarity in my activities and I am better able to serve others. This is the heart of a contemporary yoga practice. We don't need ideology or theology in order to affirm the diversity and interrelatedness of all life, but we certainly need the tools for learning how to cultivate attentiveness and to balance our internal energy patterns so that we have vitality and clarity which we can bring to the complex issues of a world out of balance.

Less than a decade into the new millennium, the world still wrestles with a plethora of problems left over from the twentieth century. There are still more than three dozen major active conflicts (those with over one thousand casualties, both military and civilian) in the world.[2] In armed conflicts since 1945, 90 percent of casualties have been civilians, compared to 50 percent in the Second World War and 10 percent in the First.[3] Three out of four fatalities of war are women and children.[4] War and internal conflicts in the 1990s forced 50 million people to flee their homes.[5] More than 500 million small arms and light weapons are in circulation around the world—one for about every twelve people.[6] These light arms were the weapons of choice in forty-six out of forty-nine major conflicts since 1990, causing four million deaths—about 90 percent of them civilians, and 80 percent women and children.[7]

Human security is under increasing threat from the spread and illegal trade of small arms and light weapons. They have devastated many societies and caused incalculable human suffering. They continue to pose an enormous humanitarian challenge, particularly in internal conflicts where insurgent militias fight against government forces. In these conflicts, a high proportion of the casualties are civilians who are the deliberate targets of violence—a gross violation of international humanitarian law. This has led to millions of deaths and injuries, the displacement of populations, and suffering and insecurity around the world.[8]

In light of these statistics, we need to once again open up the question: What is enlightenment? How can such awakening serve the great gulf of suffering that we witness when we walk through our cities or watch the news? If yoga philosophy and practice cannot answer such a question, it needs to be challenged and provoked to go beyond itself. As yoga penetrates contemporary cultures, and if its practices help awaken us, certainly we will have something to offer this ancient tradition currently coming alive in a new form; and, by extension, yoga will have something to offer this culture at this time.

We come to understand the basic unity of all things when we no longer rely on *this* and *that, inside* or *outside, black* versus *white,* and instead appreciate the complex interrelations of everything. Yoga moves us beyond our contracted viewpoint. Yoga helps us cultivate a mind that can clearly contain and enter into the wealth of sounds and colors, shapes and sizes, thoughts and sensations, and take those things back to their roots, experiencing directly the tangled roots of all experience. Kinship is everywhere, even between you and these words. When we turn to armed conflict, the first thing we notice is the way each side is contracted around a viewpoint. Again, since yoga is fueled by action, it's not that we give up all views, but that we find clarity within the passion of holding a view. The warrior Arjuna, in the epic Bhagavad Gita, must choose between passivity or war, and this leads him into deep contemplation on the nature of actions taken or not. Scholar Shashi Bhushan Dasgupta writes:

Regarding . . . the practice of the virtues of non-injury, Arjuna maintains that it is wrong to carry these virtues to extremes. Howsoever a man may live, whether as an ascetic or as a forester, it is impossible for him to practice non-injury to all living beings in any extreme degree. Even in the water that one drinks and the fruits that one eats, even in breathing and winking many fine and invisible beings are killed. So the virtue of non-injury, or, for the matter of that, all kinds of virtue, can be practiced only in moderation, and their injuctions always imply that they can be practiced only within the bounds of a common sense view of things. Non-injury may be good; but there are cases where non-injury would mean doing injury. If a tiger enters into a cattle shed, not to kill the tiger would amount to killing the cows.[9]

We spend most of each summer in sparsely populated, forested northern Ontario, where, for the last few years, the spring bear hunt has been abolished. For decades, the spring bear hunt kept the population of bears in relation to farmers and rural populations manageable, but many hunters began taking advantage of the bear-hunting regulations. Some hunters were shooting pregnant bears and others were causing terrible injury from unethical hunting practices. Ecologists have taken a strong stance against trophy-style hunting. Ecologist Mark Mathew Braunstein writes:

Hunting garners some deserved bad press. Many hunters enjoy the thrill of the kill more than the taste of the meat. What they kill, they often do not eat. A deer hunter, for instance, less likely boasts of how many pounds of meat with which the deer dressed his dining room table than of how many antler points with which the buck decorates his dining room wall. A weekend hunter who straps a dead deer atop the roof of his Lincoln Leviathan arrives home in the big city with a frozen carcass wind-beaten into inedibility.[10]

The problem with hunting, from the perspective of the yamas is that when one predator comes back from extinction, it's usually put on the game list and then hunted back into extinction. Since the bear hunt was abolished, the bears have been multiplying quickly throughout our area of Ontario. Now bears are seen almost daily and have been moving closer and closer to farmers' livestock, and often the farmers have to shoot the bears in order to protect their livestock.

When a bear was shot by our neighbor, we were outraged that a bear was shot, that we are crowding their space, that they have no food. But we were surprised to learn that its fur was turned into mittens and its meat shared with several families. Not one hair or bone was wasted. The killing of a dangerous bear became a lesson for me in the complexity of ethical responsiveness.

The absolutes of right and wrong can never be absolute, because they are alive. Truth is worth caring about because it gives meaning to our lives, but we must watch for the high moral ground and use nonviolence as a tool for connectivity and appreciation instead of divisiveness or puritanical authority. Maybe we could suggest that all hunters be responsible for eating their quarry.

We must also be careful not to idealize the natural world conceptually. Nature is not simply an extension of our psyche. The anthropomorphizing of nature robs it of its essential integrity. We cannot solve our problems by escaping from our economic, social, and ecological realities into a world of endless pastures and rivers without end. Firstly, there are few areas left on earth where rivers, plains, and forests move uninterrupted by our "progress." Stillness in the natural world most definitely brings our moral lives back from an otherwise clouded picture. By talking less and listening more, we bring forth the unshakeable realization that the natural world is our very ground of being. "One of the problems that comes with trying to take a wider view of animals," writes author Barry Lopez, "is that most of us have cut ourselves off from them conceptually. We do not think of ourselves as part of the animal kingdom."[11]

The existential integrity of humans and the natural world comes through samādhi, the complete integration of subject and object, where we gain insight into the complete contingency of "nature" and "person." From such insight, we are pressed to take action that is neither idealistic nor romantic. We must look at the relationship between sustainability and idealistic ethical principles. They must bond. The necessities of nourishing our minds and bodies and living ethically must come together in a way that creates harmony and not discord. Gary Snyder writes:

> Ahimsā taken too literally leaves out the life of the world and makes the rabbit virtuous but the hawk evil. People who must fish and hunt to live can enter into the process with gratitude and care, and no arrogant assumptions about human privilege. This cannot come from "thinking about" nature; it must come from *being* with nature.[12]

Yoga points to the natural interplay, or coupling, of the perceiver and the perceived. We are so dominated by two verbs: *to be* and *to have*. But what does action look like when we are being rather than exploiting? This question forms the core of a nonviolent attitude and our basic definition of yoga: the inherent tangled being at the base of things. Snyder cuts to the heart of the nonduality that yoga describes, and if we take this heart, nonharming is not something we do; it becomes who we are. When yoga is expressed, you *are* peace.

Every year I participate in a workshop for young people between the ages of four and eleven. We do our best not to use the term *yoga* or any other Sanskrit terms, and instead we play with language and each other in such a way that brings creative spontaneity to staff and participants alike. One of the ways we teach about interdependence is to have the kids lie down at the base of a tree and look up at the long trunk and spreading branches with the vast sky in the background. After a few minutes of giggling or fidgeting, the kids begin to appreciate the reorientation and upside-down perspective of the well-known tree. We ask them to notice the trunk and to see where the trunk ends and the branches begin. They look and look and struggle to find the edges and cannot. We do the same with the trunk and root. Where does the trunk end and the root system begin? Without talking and just through focused looking, the kids begin to see how there is no place of beginning or end. The end of the trunk is impossible to locate not because there is no trunk but because "trunk" is a name for something much larger, extending downward into everything.

After noticing the braided roots and tangled webs that we call "tree," we take this practice into other areas. We apply this insight to other people, especially our parents, in order to see how the names we have for things mask clarity of attention and complexity. Who is mother, who is father? Who are you without your name, your role, your ideas? Through this exercise we also learn about interdependence and emptiness. We see how the tree is empty of a substantial core because even the core has a core. Suddenly the eyes of the children dazzle with excitement, having discovered this for themselves with only simple suggestion.

Wisdom, in this case, is not "knowing more" but rather seeing clearly just what words are pointing toward. This allows each of us to realize both microcosm and macrocosm; to be able to see what *is* there, rather than what one hopes or expects to be there.

SOCIAL, ECOLOGICAL, SPIRITUAL

When we *are* nature, there is no longer the need to separate it out into disjointed and competing parcels of this and that. This wisdom incorporates what was there to begin with: the nonseparation of ecology, spirituality, psychology, and ethics. To incorporate is to remember to put limbs back together again, and this is exactly what comes from a well-rounded yoga practice. "This is a commitment to kinship and friendship," I often remind our extended community of practitioners, "and even when anger and war and competitiveness cross our minds, we turn kindly to those friends *also*, for we know them well." With these words we try not to divorce any part of ourselves, even the wild cast of characters that populate our minds.

Environmental degradation is as much an ecological crisis as a psychological, social, and spiritual one. As we begin to pay attention to the effects of our actions, we begin to tune in to to the meaningful place we all share in this evolving web of life. Sand dunes always change form, so do winds and tides and thought patterns; as humans living in an evolving world, we must also evolve in our imaginative response to the world's complex problems as though they were our own. Better yet, we must recognize that they are imbalances in our very self.

In terms of nonharming, we would do well to recall that ecology reminds us that organisms are the entirety of a system because those very organisms are complex ecosystems themselves. Communities of organisms are made up of smaller sets of organisms in the same way those in prison are intertwined with those outside. From the beginning, ecology is defined by interdependence, complementary opposites, and cooperation. The web of human activity thus requires nonharming as a central principle, or else we will set up patterns that split and divide the body here, there, and everywhere. At bottom, there is no separation.

NEW PATHWAYS

It is not possible to use nonviolence, in the truest sense, to accomplish a violent end. Any duality between good and evil is ultimately delusive since good depends on evil and evil is contingent on the category of good. Can we open up to more flexible modes of perception?

The year 2006 ended with the execution of Saddam Hussein. Photographs of his execution spread like wildfire across the Internet and by the end of the news day, images of Saddam Hussein were on every newsstand. His actual death and, of course, its symbolic value equate revenge with justice and perpetuate the ongoing momentum of violence, not only in the news media but in our innermost being. Can we put yogic principles to work on the execution of Saddam Hussein?

Yoga is about the nondual nature of reality. When we hang Sadaam Hussein, we are giving credence to killing as a valid response to violence.

Does this form of punishment annul the crimes against humanity? To punish is to harm, and the intent to harm sets up the conditions for future aggression and violence. Can we instead approach punishment with the wisdom of nondual psychology? How can our relationships—all of them—be just and peaceful? When injustice and violence occur, how can we respond by restoring peace and decency rather than responding to violence with violence? How can we move toward the conditions that give rise to violence and take them apart, investigate them, and respond in a way that ends the cycle of injury and anger?

Conflict is inevitable. Aggression is inevitable. Violence will occur as long as we are the people we are—humans are always born into this world with ancestral habit energies that need attention, redirection, and transformation. The principles that create or deny peace are the same in our relationships with friends and lovers, our relationships with our cultural attitudes and ourselves. Maybe how we have dealt with Saddam Hussein is a barometer of our lack of creative and peaceful means for dealing with violence and injustice? Is there another way?

The main cause of evil in our current global culture may, in fact, be our attempts to eradicate evil. Even the spectacular white of the moon hides a shadow. The shadows in us that we cannot accept constrain our freedom. What we cannot accept we cannot be free of. We are a community of individuals, not concepts competing with one another; if we can't begin to accept others and understand their position, even their anger, there is no possibility of yoga.

We all want security and freedom. Execution does not guarantee either of these. When we act out of fear, we find ourselves as alienated "selves" threatened by the world and seeking security from anxiety. Can we better understand Saddam Hussein's anxiety, and, even if not, can we attend to the conditions—social, economic, religious—that produce Saddam Hussein? A nondual self knows itself to be a manifestation of community. Saddam Hussein *is* our community.

What is war or assassination doing for us? If it is not satisfying something in us, we would not continue. What is being satisfied in our obsession with war? If war is one way of dealing with lack, how can we ever be free? The statistics during the US-led mission in Iraq describe a population confused and apathetic. Even after official inquiries have completely undermined government and media propaganda about Saddam's weapons of mass destruction and links to Al-Qaeda, half the United States population continue to believe the charges, and thus support not only the invasion—the "supreme international crime differing only from other war crimes in that it contains within itself the accumulated evil of the whole," in the wording of the Nuremberg Tribunal—but also the ongoing war crimes directed by United States forces[13] that are depicted without shame on the front pages of the world's popular newspapers, always in self-defense against evil forces threatening us with destruction. We cannot underestimate the threat of terror or the cynicism of centers of power in pursuit of their own often despicable ends or the murderous violence to which they will resort if authority is granted to them by a frightened population. Meanwhile families on both sides post bulletins of the lost, missing, and wounded. Children are anxious.

When we react out of fear and hatred, we do not yet have a deep understanding of the situation. Our actions will only be a very quick and superficial way of responding to the state of affairs, and not much true benefit and healing will occur. Yet if we wait and follow the process of calming our anger, looking deeply into the situation, and listening with great will to understand the roots of suffering that are the cause of the violent actions, only then will we have sufficient insight to respond in such a way that healing and reconciliation can be realized for everyone involved. This is hard work and, in some ways, counterintuitive. The prevailing attitude of putting up a strong fight promotes invincibility, not communication. Such an attitude makes listening very difficult for both sides and obviously makes the trust necessary for changing opinion almost impossible. As much as we want yoga teachings to tell us what to do in the face of war, they cannot. But they can, of course, realign our attitude so that we can freely contribute to the welfare of others and see beyond our clinging and aggression. Any long-term corrective to the arising of terror and violence must grow out of a commitment to refining and reimagining the quality and meaning of relationships—our individual and collective patterns of interdependence.

THE PRACTICAL ANTIDOTE

Love and listening are the antidotes to fear. Generosity sets up the conditions for letting go. Rather than repeating the same habits over and over, we can bring to our intolerance and inflexibility a deep appreciation for our creativity and the capacity to reimagine conflict from the ground of nonharming. Certainly, in the face of fear, what we need most is flexibility in our cultural imagination, rather than fixed categories of good or the inflated and dangerous ideal of ridding the world of evil. Can we turn to others not with habitual consolation or empathic technique but with the embodied manner of service and generosity? Don't we all share something in common?

A student of mine who works as a diplomat in Gaza, trying to keep the borders open between Israel and Egypt, described her impossible profession in these words:

> None of us can get any work done. We spin in circles. We have no idea how to take action because we have no idea how to listen. We think we can listen but we have lost the skills. We are too stuck in our viewpoints to hear anything the other side has to say.

On retreat together, we practiced meditating on sound, both individually and in groups. We spent time quietly listening. We called this "listening without knowing." Sometimes we sat up, sometimes we walked, and sometimes we lay around, but we were always attentive. We worked in pairs, slowly trying to listen to what others have to say, staying with our breathing, feeling the body, and allowing each other to speak without interruption. Then we practiced speaking our viewpoint and allowing others to do the same without finishing each others' sentences or contracting in the body. It was a powerful week that reminded all of us how the same skills that we apply in our own minds reverberate as skills in the collective domain. Practice inside moves outside, and the outside is reworked internally. "Now go back to work," I said to her at the end of the retreat, to which she responded, "Now I see the work I have to do, and it's much simpler than I ever thought." I didn't really understand the complexity of Egyptian-Israeli politics, and I still know very little, but I was amazed at what a difference listening made in the minds and hearts of these diplomats.

When Saddam Hussein barred UN inspectors from visiting alleged chemical and biological weapons sites in Iraq, the Clinton administration responded with a swift military build-up in the Persian Gulf. Although most of the international community strongly opposed a military solution to the crisis, the United States repeatedly stated that it would act unilaterally if necessary. Only Britain, which dispatched an aircraft carrier to the area, offered unwavering support for a military strike.

From military build-up to terrorism or torture, is there another way we can respond to such threats? "Torture," from Gandhi's point of view, "is ineffective . . . because it corrupts the moral character of a society that allows it to be used."[14]

Gandhi also felt that cowardice was more violent than raw anger and spoke strongly against the belief that peace is impossible. In one of his most famous remarks on the topic, during a conversation with someone who was providing tepid responses to complex issues, Gandhi said: "When there is only a choice between cowardice and violence, I would advise violence."[15] Gandhi often gave the example of meeting a mad dog with rabies and acting swiftly and immediately by either maiming or killing it. "Inaction at the time of conflagration is inexcusable," he said.[16]

Gandhi's approach is to take action specific to the circumstances while maintaining the reality of relational existence, extending our capacity to listen indefinitely. That violence begets violence cannot be overstated. Furthermore, Gandhi's first steps were always communication and flexibility. Gandhi made solutions possible through the act of listening. He embodied nonharming, because his intent was not fear-based but rather honest and open—qualities that promote relationship and dialogue, creating solutions that both sides can accept in part because both sides are given attention and respect. We must still face the difficult task of putting our values to work in our lives, families, and communities, always working with the thorny issues of this time.

From the perspective of yoga, the real question behind the execution of Saddam Hussein is one that is both psychological and social: Can we begin to see how the duality between good and evil is ultimately delusive? Can we move to a more insightful mode of investigation where we can acknowledge that peace involves not just looking into good and evil philosophically but rather understanding the relationship between love and fear?

The fruit of the yoga path, and perhaps that of all religions and spiritual disciplines, is the end of a life organized by fear. Stephen Batchelor, writing on the topic of the September 11 attacks, says:

> [If a practitioner] regards all sentient beings as "us," then he or she cannot treat even those who hijack civilian aircraft and turn them into guided missiles as "them." However difficult, we have to be able to empathize not only with their victims but also with the terrorists themselves. Condemning acts as evil does not entail condemning the people who committed them as evil. One has to try to understand the origins of their suffering and the reasons that led them to commit appalling acts of violence. It is probable that the men who flew the planes into the twin towers and the Pentagon believed that they were doing good, possibly out of sincere religious motives.[17]

Then he goes on to say:

But each of us is to some extent implicated in contributing to the conditions from which these acts of violence arose. By tolerating the way our governments behave abroad, by making investments in the corporations that sustain the global economy, by consuming fossil fuels, we are complicit in the intricate web of relationships that sustains the world as it is. The sheer complexity, scale and speed of these interactions can make one feel utterly confused and powerless. The challenge is to respond to that confusion without lapsing into the oppositional rhetoric of "us" versus "them" or retreating to a mystical equanimity that trusts that everything is part of a divine plan or the working out of karmic consequences beyond our individual comprehension.[18]

Our challenge is to clarify the difference between reactions and responses, and to act from a place of commitment to a longer-term vision of nonviolence. There are many different types of crimes committed by many different types of people in all kinds of varied situations. But we can always approach these various contexts with as open a view as possible yet matched, however difficult it seems at times, with an attitude of peace. Napoléon is supposed to have remarked that one can do anything with bayonets except sit on them. We can always sow the seeds of peace even when our listening faculties are shutting down in the face of fear. Do not turn away. Our practice reminds us to not turn away. Equanimity grows out of a compassion for everyone involved when one person hurts another. In his essay on the Bhagavad Gita and its story line in the context of the violent Mahabharata, Gandhi writes: "The author of the Mahabharata has not established the necessity of physical warfare; on the contrary, he has proved its futility. He has made the victors shed tears of sorrow and repentance, he has left them nothing but a legacy of miseries."[19]

All violence is injustice, but let's be careful where we create opposition between what is happening and what we think ought not to happen. Somewhere between what is actually occurring and our concepts about what is occurring, we find a rich and fertile zone of possibility. We need to leave behind the place where our ideas get in the way of seeing the complexity and interdependence of a given situation. The fire of hatred and violence cannot be extinguished by adding more hatred and violence as fuel. The only antidote to violence is compassion.

Nonviolence begins with how we choose to perceive each given circumstance. Anger is nothing other than a smoke screen for fear. Saddam Hussein inflicted terrible violence in his lifetime, but we do not have to respond to his violence with actions that set up the condition for further violence.

The more we try to control things, the more disorder is created. What kind of society do we want to live in?

CHAPTER SIX

SATYA: HONESTY

Focusing with perfect discipline on friendliness,
compassion, delight and equanimity, one is imbued
with their energies.

—PATAÑJALI, *Yoga-Sūtra*

You don't see the center of the universe
because it's all center.

—C. S. LEWIS

S ATYA, AS A term and practice, is the most straightforward of the
yamas. The word itself is derived from the root *sat* meaning "to be."
Being is not passive, because we are always in action. As we mature and
move about the world determining what makes most sense to us, we are
always confronted with idioms and options, character possibilities, and
the always rising push of desire.

Usually the term "satya" is translated as "truthfulness," though I
prefer the word "honesty" to "truth" because "truth" can be conceptual,
overly objective, and oftentimes dogmatic. Honesty is more subjective,
personally authentic and of collective value. Living honestly is more
than just understanding how things work or having good philosophical

ideas. We can see truthful living in simple farmers that is sometimes lacking in people with wealth; we can see truthful living in young people that is sometimes lacking in their parents.

Like the other principles of restraint, honesty (satya) challenges us to focus our awareness on the relationship between the actions of our body, speech, and mind and the effects of these actions individually and across the human, human-built, and nonhuman spectra. Can attention to honesty be a strategy by which we can wake up to interconnectedness and act from a place of friendliness, compassion, delight, and equanimity? Can we apply the yama of honesty to every aspect of our personal and cultural lives, from how we speak with others to how we determine how much we really need?

HONESTY AND DESIRE

The yamas begin a yogic diagnosis and remedy for the human condition in terms of our understanding of contemporary society, and honesty—satya—goes a long way in helping us see clearly. As we still the distractions of mind and body and settle into a more authentic way of being in and of the world, we also awake to a larger responsibility, namely, serving and supporting others where they are suffering. Yoga practice brings about the unshakable realization that everything is empty of self-image and that, at bottom, the personality is a relational matrix. If we are all interconnected—an insight common during stillness and silence—we come to see that the choices we make have a significant effect on the overall well-being of others. But who is the other? Is the other only that which is not me? Where and how do I create the division? Furthermore, let's not fall into the trap of thinking "other" refers only to humans.

Like other world religions and spiritual practices, yoga has traditionally been limited by very simplistic social theories and assumptions. Only comparatively recently has society become sufficiently dynamic and complex to stimulate the development of an adequately responsive and explanatory social and ecological theory. From the time of our birth, we each respond not only in a personal sense to the precariousness of our human condition, but we are also the inheritors of delusive social institutions and shared meanings about the world. The same basic patterns we find in our minds and bodies are also found in the structure and function of our institutions.[1]

The environmental damage that industry is causing across the American landscape is usually described by environmentalists as a problem with "them," with industry. Jonathan Porritt, an eloquent communicator of environmental policy, writes:

> Interestingly, however, [cause and blame are] rarely pointed at individual citizens: it's the politicians that represent them, or the businesses that provide for their every want or need, that are put on the dock. When did you last hear an environmental organization castigate ordinary people in the UK for leading such greedy, self-obsessed, unhealthy, lazy, indifferent or even callous lives? Or (to be a bit more positive about it!), what percentage of the total spending deployed by environmental organizations in the UK is devoted to changing people's behaviors rather than changing the minds of legislators or business leaders?[2]

One of the most important issues on which we can put satya to work is the issue of personal and collective consumption and our skewed ideas about what we need. Today's consumption is undermining the environmental resource base. It is exacerbating inequalities and causing irreparable damage to the body of the world. The dynamics of the consumption-poverty-inequality-environment nexus are accelerating. If these trends continue without change—not redistributing wealth from high-income to low-income citizens, not shifting from pollutants to cleaner goods and production technologies, not promoting goods that empower poor producers, not shifting priority from consumption for conspicuous display to consumption for meeting basic needs—today's problems of consumption and human development will worsen. So too will terrorism and the kind of violence that occurs when groups are marginalized by these kinds of consumption patterns and the worldview that informs them.

As we've discussed in terms of karma, the real issue is not consumption itself but its patterns and effects. Inequalities in consumption are stark. People in the world's high-income countries account for 81.5 percent of total private consumption expenditures—people in the world's low-income countries account for just 3.6 percent.[3]

We consume a variety of resources and products today, having moved beyond basic needs to include luxury items and technological innovations that try to improve efficiency. Such consumption beyond minimal and basic needs is not necessarily a bad thing in and of itself, as throughout history we have always sought to find ways to make our lives a bit easier to live. However, increasingly, there are important issues around consumerism that need to be understood. In a recent yoga retreat aimed at exploring the relationship between yoga postures, meditation, philosophy, and the environment, a group of us came up with a list of questions that would help us see our consumption patterns with greater clarity and honesty. Here's what we came up with:

· How are the products and resources we consume actually produced?
· What are the impacts of that process of production on the environment, society, and individuals?
· What are the impacts of certain forms of consumption on the environment, on society, and on individuals?
· Which factors influence our choices of consumption?
· Which factors influence how and why things are produced or not?
· What is a necessity, and what is a luxury?
· How do consumption habits change as the values of societies change?

Businesses and advertising are major engines in promoting the consumption of products for their own survival. We could add to this list questions such as: How much of what we consume is influenced by their needs versus our needs? What is the impact on poorer nations and people from the demands of the wealthier nations and people that are able to afford to consume more? How do material values influence our relationships with other people? What impact does this have on our personal values? What do we really need?

Just from these questions, we can likely think of numerous others as well. Additionally, we can see that consumerism and consumption are at the core of many, if not most, societies. The impacts of consumerism, positive and negative, are very significant to all aspects of our lives, as well as our planet. But equally important to bear in mind in discussing consumption patterns is the underlying system that promotes certain types of consumption and not other types.

Inherent in today's global economic system is the wasteful use of resources, labor, and capital. This needs to be addressed. It's disturbing how many people are engaged in work that they feel is not worthwhile. Our skills and joy for work are often repressed by the demands of our own greed, fast pace, and inattention to what matters. What are we trying to overcome or fill when we can't or don't want to see the nexus of our values, moods, and consumption patterns? Duḥkha and consumption are intimately related.

When we try to respond to these questions, the effects of our actions are hard-hitting and highlight one of the major impacts of today's form of corporate-led globalization. Overpopulation is usually blamed as the major cause of environmental degradation, but statistics strongly suggest otherwise. Consumption patterns today are not indicative of everyone's needs. The planet simply cannot sustain our obsession with converting more and more resources into accumulating more and more overpackaged and useless products. The system that drives these consumption patterns also contributes to the inequality of consumption patterns. The "system," however, is you and I.

Consuming things we don't need or sometimes don't even want offers the dissatisfied mind a temporary and elusive grasp on reality. When our lives are motivated by a desire to find security in external objects or to ground ourselves through the accumulation of wealth, we lose touch with the fact that these superficial symbols are only representations of what is important. What needs are such purchases trying to fill? The reality of our spiritual hunger shines through statistics of global inequality and the wealth-poverty divide. What are we hungry for?

Freud reminds us that anything we repress comes back to us in the form of a symptom. A symptom is therefore a symbolic representation of something repressed or underexpressed, something that we are trying to exclude from consciousness. Any form of repression creates discord and imbalance. If we look into the symptoms within and around us—overconsumption, aggression, greed, envy, the desire for fame, for romantic love—we see how our spiritual hunger appears in symptom form. What we seek outside of us illustrates what we think we lack.

The preoccupation with material things seen daily in every shopping mall illustrates our skewed efforts to deal with the basic existential question of having been born into a life structured by death. Our absolute devotion to accumulation and security masks something deep in the formation of the personality, namely, the fact that the self will never be satisfied because it does not exist as something separate in the first place.

To forget ourselves in moments of creativity and to ultimately let go of the compulsive activity of constructing a separate self means finding ourselves immersed in the world. The present ecological and social crises across the world testify to the importance of responding to the world as being intimately tied to every aspect of our basic nature. Yoga provides us with a guideline for how to live in the world as if it was our very self, because at bottom that is exactly how nature operates. There is no separation. A body of water cannot vote and neither can a rain forest. Yoga challenges us to move into the world guided by nonviolent means and remain grounded in a spiritual practice rooted in honest and responsive action. This means examining our attachments and how they affect our worldview. Even with new developments in environmental policy, we need to include the possibility of renunciation, or we'll continue to believe that one ton of carbon over here is actually balanced by trading one ton of carbon over there. It's hard to see clearly when we are pushed and pulled by the unexamined assumption that nature's seemingly infinite storehouse is there for us to use without let or hindrance for whatever purposes we see fit. It's hard to see clearly when we are entangled in our endless preoccupations and insatiable wants.

TIME

In the contemporary world, poverty is caused by the growth and maintenance of ownership in large concentrations that take from society more than they give. Most of the wealth that is concentrated in elite hands has been accumulated through the hard work of others. Consumerism supports this cycle and robs us of precious time. Time is exchanged for money to buy things and then there is less and less time to enjoy. We spend our time working for things, and in the little time we have to relax, we spend that time in front of the television where we watch mediocre filler programs inserted in between ever more spectacular commercials whose purpose is to create more desire for more things—that we have to work longer hours to purchase. By robbing us of time, consumerism has a deleterious effect on family life. Stephen Batchelor writes:

> Today . . . as we live and work in a world of . . . great complexity, where the apparently simple acts of buying and selling have repercussions on people's lives around the world, the ethics of right livelihood must be accordingly reevaluated. The implications of even driving a car or drinking a cup of coffee have social, environmental, and economic consequences far beyond the limits of our immediate experience, which we are morally obligated to

take into account. From this perspective, inner spiritual transformation is just as dependent upon the effect of our economic life
upon the world as transformations in the world are dependent
upon spiritual re-orientation.[4]

HONESTY, CONTENTMENT, AND PEACE

In exploring the five yamas we are, in essence, discovering a path toward peace. Yoga is a path of peacemaking. "Peace" is a word that is
uttered almost as frequently as "truth," "beauty," and "love," and may be
just as elusive to define as these other virtues. Common synonyms for
peace include "amity," "friendship," "harmony," "concord," "tranquility,"
"repose," "quiescence," "truce," "pacification," and "neutrality." Likewise,
the peacemaker is the pacifier, mediator, intermediary, and intercessor.
While some of these descriptions are appropriate for conflict resolu-
tion, they are still quite limited in describing both the nature of peace
and the role of the peacemaker in moment-to-moment living. Any
attempt to articulate the nature of peace and peacemaking, therefore,
must address those conditions that are favorable to their emergence.
The ground of those conditions is satya, honesty, and an attention span
not bound by ideology or fixed views. This is not to say we have no
viewpoint. When we watch our minds and bodies from a place of stillness, we come to see that as objects of consciousness move through
awareness, the mind does not have to stick to one thing or another,
and, when the mind does not dwell on "this" or "that," a final view
or opinion is not a completion point but rather another mental moment in an infinite arc of thought. We are a culture with an acute form
of attention deficit disorder, and to recognize the inherent stillness in
all movement, we need to embark on a practice that teaches us how
to work with the tendency to contract around each and every state of
mind, emotion, or sensation.

For peace to emerge, we must respect the rights of other people, species, and living things. Respect requires not only honest appraisal but

also the ability to allow ourselves to be changed by that which we are experiencing. Other prerequisites for peace include sensitivity to injustice and the proactive energy that comes from seeing injustice and feeling its effects. Peace begins by not turning away from suffering.

Our culture holds violence in high status—just look at any news channel, radio report, or newspaper (or indeed any conflict in the home) to see the nature of anger, aggression, and violence in ourselves and in one another.

The yamas circle around one primary question: Why is human open-mindedness continually diminished and evaded? Why does egoism retain such a stronghold even when our intention to benefit others gains momentum? This begs a further question, namely: Why is our capacity to be flexible, to see all living beings as equal, and to act out of that insight in honesty and intimacy with all things so rarely exercised? What are we defending when we create a self that falls into comfort, habit, and prejudice more easily than open-mindedness and intimacy?

It is not enough to simply still the mind or see through the always-present strategies of self-image; we must actually transform these states of mind into a genuine care for others and the world at large. Our longing is satisfied not with things external to us but out of the clarifying practice of the yamas—attentiveness to the way that our entire existence is built through and from relationship.

Yoga is a release from preoccupation with ourselves and that release is sometimes joyous and other times painful. We cling to our history even when our history is painful. We cling to bad habits even when we know otherwise. We always desire what is known and comfortable even when it's bad for us if only because it's a repeatable experience— predictable, comfortable, conservative. This conservative and repetitive aspect of the human personality is exactly what the yamas and all yogic practices focus on interrupting. Reality is always greater than our theories of reality, and the unbound attention the yamas orient us toward brightens and clarifies the yogic way.

OPENING UP AND SHUTTING DOWN

Satya is the honest recollection of our lives, the honest meeting of each moment, the honest lovemaking with one's partner, and the honest gaze of satisfied eyes. Honesty is not looking away from suffering, or from any moment in the ongoing vicissitude of experience. Honesty should not be misconstrued as a way of living that takes the difficulty out of being truthful—this is a challenging path. To be honest in speech, to honestly look at the mind and our habits of deception is no small enterprise, and the path of yoga encourages a path without escape. "I think speaking truthfully is a more fitting ambition that speaking the truth," writes psychology theorist Leslie Faber.[5] Like Patañjali's image as both a stainless white serpent and a human being, we have in all of us the capacity to wake up, act honestly, and make choices from a place of compassion; yet, we also have the opposite tendency: to shut down, return to our habitual grooves, and act out of our most unconscious habits. Faber continues, "It is in our nature to lie, but I think I must add that it is also in our nature not to lie."[6] Faber moves close to the heart of what it means to be human. Like Patañjali's paradoxical body, our capacities to wake up and to shut down, and the back-and-forth bellowslike movement between the two, become the work of our spiritual path. At all platforms along the way (and in every chapter of his *Yoga-Sūtra*), Patañjali warns of the ways that the self comes to hijack our practice. "Self-clinging is perpetual," Patañjali warns, "even for the wise."[7] Honesty is the act of intersecting and eventually dissecting the hypnotic quality of cheating, deceiving, and lying. Honesty serves the basic principle of not causing harm. Honesty plucks from our actions the intention to cause harm.

Like the other yamas, we are dealing here with what is realistic, not some idealized version of oneself that can create just another trap of self-image. When we move from a place of clear seeing and take actions in such a way that we are not intentionally causing harm to ourselves or others, all that is left is to entrust ourselves to intimacy. Honesty demands that we look after each other for no other reason than the fact of our interconnectedness. If you and I are essentially yoked, how could being dishonest be beneficial? Since honesty arrives in Patañjali's list just after nonharming, honesty must always be tempered by nonharm so that we are attentive to the power of communication and its consequences.

In 1906, feeling that he needed a better description of the kind of work he was pursuing through his activism and writing, Gandhi asked his readers to contribute terms that best suited his struggle. Gandhi's journal *Indian Opinion* was extraordinarily popular among activists and citizens alike, and he used the wide reach of his journal to explore what terms might best describe his method. His cousin Maganlal came up with the idea of using the term "the force of truth." Gandhi refined the term by integrating the second yama, "satya," with the fifth, "āgraha," to create the neologism "satyagraha," which means "grasping truth" or "holding honesty." "Āgraha" means "holding something firmly," and for Gandhi, nonviolent action begins with satyagraha, holding firmly to the honest approach. Scholar Mark Juergensmeyer writes,

> What Gandhi found appealing about the winning phrase was its focus on truth. Gandhi reasoned that no one possesses a complete view of it. The very existence of a conflict indicates a deep difference over what is right. The first task of a conflict, then, is to try to see the conflict from both sides of the issue.[8]

Communication enlarges our vision of truth. Since our perception is limited, honesty requires that with patience and flexibility we begin to allow possibilities to arise before we make a decision in the belief that we are following truth. What Gandhi is saying through the yama of satya is that truth is always partial; like violence, dishonesty is inevitable, yet through attention and sensitivity, wisdom arises through our mistakes.

A shared cultural commitment to honesty supports a culture of awakening. Personal psychology informs culture, and a culture of nonviolence changes the way we think and perceive. We cannot separate

personal and social spheres when it comes to ethical and spiritual awakening. After the terrible abuse of prisoners at the American prison at
Abu Ghraib in Iraq, many people wondered whether it was the fault
of the US military or the individual soldiers themselves. Beginning in
2004, accounts of abuse, torture, rape, and homicide of prisoners held
in the Abu Ghraib prison in Iraq (also known as Baghdad Central
Correctional Facility) came to public attention. The acts were committed by some personnel of the 372nd Military Police Company of the
United States, and possibly additional American governmental agen-
cies. As revealed by the 2004 Taguba Report, a criminal investigation
by the US Army Criminal Investigation Command had already been
under way since 2003 and multiple recruits from the 320th Military
Police Battalion had been charged under the Uniform Code of Military Justice with prisoner abuse. In 2004, articles of the abuse, including
pictures showing military personnel abusing prisoners, came to public
attention when a *60 Minutes* news report (on April 28) and an article
by Seymour M. Hersh in *The New Yorker* magazine (posted online on
April 30 and published days later in the May 10 issue) reported the
story. The soldiers knew that violence did not help gather intelligence,
and the kind of violence American soldiers pursued with the prisoners was sexual humiliation, not physical beating or hitting. When we
keep locating the violence "out there," Homeland security becomes a
righteous belief that our land is separate from the kind of violence one
sees in Iraq. But the truth of the matter, especially as illustrated by the
treatment of Iraqi prisoners, tells a very different story. Our psychological homeland is literally our belief systems. Homeland security begins
with honesty about the state of our psychological homeland. We *are* our
actions.

False words have no meaning. If words have no meaning and are not
connected through one another via mind, body, and heart, they have no
power to connect and affect change within a community. We cannot
build community when there is dishonesty in our hearts. Building an
ecological culture of yoga begins with love. In such a culture people ex-

pend themselves in love and work because those whom they love have a value beyond time and beyond human understanding. We work on projects that outlive us, and in such actions we redefine ourselves in a web and span much greater than our short personal histories.

Since belief precedes actions, we need to be honest about where our beliefs are narrow, dogmatic, or violent. This is hard to do because our core beliefs are usually quite unconscious. We all harbor more biases than we might think. When I meet someone on the street, I can judge their dress, skin color, health, level of mobility, gender, and many other categories within a split second. From there, another split second makes association to these categories: she is poor, he is single, she is lazy, they are rude, and so on. In the blink of an eye, emotional prejudice seeps into our first beliefs about someone, and as an impulse activity it is automatic.

To survive we need to know what we are looking at, but the way that the brain constructs contexts is often wrong or outdated. Learning to deal with differences is very difficult, and trying to overcome prejudice is much harder. The practice of the yamas, supported by meditation practice, allows us to see the relationship between our beliefs, the choices we make, the consequences of our actions, and the reactivity and fear in the mind that often leads to prejudice. Is it possible to look and listen without knowing?

A student at our center recently returned from overseas, where he had been reporting on a young suicide bomber who caused tremendous devastation when he walked onto a bus with a vest of explosives that was detonated from a safe distance by a cellular telephone. The reporter, who is new to meditative practices, described how when he listened to what the innocent civilians who were injured had to say and also what the families of the perpetrators had to say, he had no idea who was "right" or "wrong." "It's not that the devastation wasn't horrific," he said, "or that I was in shock myself. I *was* a mess. But I also found that I've been trained as a reporter to find a good story. Since I was so distressed by the amount of violence I've reported on, I decided to implement the meditative practices we've been working on. And what I found was that when I listened to both sides without memory or too much knowing, I realized both sides were in pain. And something happened where I wanted to reach out to both sides, who, in their own strange ways, wanted peace, wanted a simple and harmonious life."

Not knowing—giving up fixed ideas about ourselves and others—begins where familiar ways of knowing come to an end. When we let go of the enclosures that come with set beliefs, when we find flexibility through the renunciation of our favorite viewpoints, we refuse being drawn into the binary box of "us" and "them." This is where the recognition of the web of life begins. When there are fewer seams between "me" and "you," borders become relative and communication begins. Free from the turbulence of a mind spinning with rights and wrongs, we can let go in the spaciousness of awareness. This is the path of yoga.

People always gravitate to what is familiar because it is known. Yoga pushes us to move beyond these categories by stressing actions that come from honest appraisal, a commitment to nonviolence, and a deep trust in not clinging to views. The path of satya, when successful, results in greater freedom, which is a mode of being rather than a particular act of renunciation. Satya is the effect of committed practice and the expression of our realization in active life.

Practitioners always need to address this question: How does this practice make its expression through the activity of my life?

Satya is the honest examination of the fabric of our relational lives and the uncontrived expression of our realization of that particular fabric. In revealing life with clarity and authenticity, the tools of satya, like the other yamas, open the doorway of compassion. Satya is not something you do out of religious faith in doctrine, but a way we express in each and every moment a deep commitment and care to the web of life of which we are only a part. This realization forms the ground and entire path of yoga practice. Maple leaves, the rooster at dawn, the pol-

luting paper mill, sands on the bank of a river, walking with a friend—
these are not enclosed instances or separate activities important only
in their individual worlds; they are the expression of life taking its
course, moving through each and every part of the web, and they are
sustained by the web itself. Each "thing" has it own suchness (tattva),
yet it is fundamentally equal with everything else. A conversation with
a friend has as much right to exist as the little ant passing through our
shared meal.

As a twelve-year-old girl, Ruth Klüger was imprisoned in a concentration camp. When a selection was made in the women's camp to
segregate women between the ages of fifteen and forty-five for a labor
camp—and labor meant, at least, continuing to live—the girl had difficulty giving her age other than her true one. When she had already
been rejected, which would have meant her certain death, her mother
begged her to try again with another SS selection officer, giving an in-
correct age. She then resolved to claim that she was already thirteen!
Only when a female guard assisting the SS man whispered to her that
she should say she was fifteen did she actually do so.[9]

Transgressing certain prohibitions challenges us to contemplate
morality. It requires a letting go of our assumptions and, as discussed
throughout this book, our attachments—responding immediately in a
situation as that situation requires. Rules can't help. What are we going
to do?

OPTIMUM BALANCE

We should be optimistic. All systems find their ongoing health, complexity, and vitality through overcoming threats to their balance and
harmony. A forest fire brings new life to the forest floor, and the personal crises we all face during certain phases of life bring renewal and
wisdom. This world is too large and diverse for any ideology that creates constriction or orthodoxy. Turning to the historical teachings of

yoga is an attempt to provide guidelines for our current forms of action and methods for working with the mind, but not an idealization of an ancient culture in an age so different than ours. Yoga is not a system that should be treated as the last word, but rather an attempt to create a platform upon which we can build a thoughtful and coherent response to our current individual, collective, and ecological problems.

When we are caught up in denial, our perceptual abilities are obscured. We should not underestimate the power of grounded observation, or bearing witness. The first step of yoga is to start where we are, and this usually means recognizing where there is discontent or suffering. When we begin with the truth of suffering both in the human, nonhuman, and human-built realms, we begin to move out of the denial or apathy that most cultural media perpetuates. When Rachel Carson published *Silent Spring* in 1962, she sent shock waves through a culture caught up in unconscious denial. Carson articulated the effects of our actions, and her work is still causing change. What Carson inspired was a movement not based on theory or political ideology, but on a simple articulation of what she saw. And what did she see?

When Carson stepped out into the fields and communities affected by toxic pesticides, when she looked at the chain of agriculture producing toxicity in the land and in humans, she didn't look away nor did she attempt to create a grand theory that promised solutions. *Silent Spring* was an achievement of observation—the willingness to be honest about what she saw. When denial is present, when the mind is caught up in habit energies, when we are not mindful, we move on automatic pilot and we do not see the consequences of our actions.

HONESTY AND COMMUNITY PRACTICE

Being honest in how we speak makes room for listening, and listening creates space in the mind's contracted habits. Shakespeare's Polonius tells us:

> This above all,
> to thine own self be true,
> and it must follow, as the night the day,
> thou canst not then be false to any man.[10]

Honesty and authenticity go hand in hand, and when they do, especially over sustained periods, our actions, ethics, and the effect of our
practice in the larger word begin to intertwine. Psychological change,
dethroning the self-making project, and taking ethical action are complementary endeavors. When we are dishonest with other people, we
are not at all in relationship with them or ourselves but rather in a
fiction built on further fiction. This inauthenticity leaves us alienated.
Personal authenticity is always constructed in the context of relationship, because we are never finished. Just as these words are shared by
you and were invented by people long before I typed them or thought
them, our personality is just a continual and contingent unfolding
without end.

Sometimes it's hard for people to grasp the complex agenda of our
practice community in Toronto, Centre of Gravity Sangha. We don't
operate as a commercial yoga studio, we are not a temple, and we have
no affiliations with any movement. Though we have strong ties to the
academic and medical communities through research and teaching
initiatives, we have remained grassroots and democratic even as we've
grown.

Centre of Gravity Sangha is an anarchic experiment of sincere
practitioners interested in the integration of contemplative practice
and daily life without the trappings of an institutionalized practice atmosphere. We have no membership structure and classes are offered
through donation. Our courses, classes, and retreats integrate formal
meditation, yoga āsana, silence, and community outreach programs.

The thrust of our practice is to support a culture of awakening by
doing the following:

1. Returning to yoga practice its tantric and nondual roots by cultivating a yoga practice that aims to concentrate the mind, wake up the intelligence of the body, and decenter the habit energies that create a separate sense of self.

2. Combining a commitment to practice and a critical engagement with the basic tenets of yoga, especially the teachings of karma and ahimsā so that our practice is put to use in everyday life.

3. Expanding our understanding of community beyond the borders of a particular school or lineage, even beyond the human realm, so that "sangha" refers to the entire web of life. This brings with it an obligation of responsible action within the web.

4. Ensuring that our practice leaves no stone unturned by practicing ethical principles, breathing therapeutics, yoga postures, meditation, and integration. A strong formal practice gives us the skills necessary for recognizing the inherent yoga in everything and in all that we do.

5. Ensuring, through personal mentorship in the form of interviews and group interaction, that we don't hide in our practice and that we continually realize practice through true self-expression.

As we cultivate equanimity and kindness, friendliness and joy, within our communities and ourselves, we counteract the ill will, jealousy, or envy that are the foundation for a competitive culture. Leaving competition behind, we can enjoy each other in similarity and in difference. Even in this consumer-driven culture, we can be motivated to improve our circumstances without resenting those who already have wealth or privilege. Similarly, we can see our own economic situation in light of others' misfortune or poverty without looking down on them. We can accept that people have accumulated different tendencies and have different abilities.

The law of karma reminds us that our health and economic situation is the product of many past actions, yet our situation can change in any moment. Acceptance is not indifference; it is the ability to return to a

place of stillness, to be nonreactive, and to weigh things carefully. This is
an important quality especially when considering social action or social
responsibility. Without acceptance and equanimity, we can get drawn
into our own reactiveness and contraction around views. The ability to
listen but also to protest is the heart of social action, the root of structural change, and the oxygen of democracy.

We'd all like to practice meditation with our legs crossed in some
clearing along a quiet river. But our formal practice, no matter how perfect, is always happening within a wider, changing world—a world that
demands our attention especially now that we've modified the natural
world to such a great degree. Even though we breathe as plants do and
live from water, we don't always see how threatening the ecological balance of the planet threatens our own bodies. A human-altered world
is making identification with the wild more and more difficult. Since
human health depends on nature's health, and since the natural world is
now dependent on our activities, we need to turn back to this body and
reconnect with its basic operations.

Inner and outer peace must be seen in terms of their interrelations
in the same way that the tightening reciprocal relationship between human health and the natural world drives home the importance of interdependence. Peace is a state of well-being that is characterized by trust,
compassion, and justice. In this state, we can be encouraged to explore
as well as celebrate our diversity, and search for the good in each other
without the concern for personal pain and sacrifice. It provides us a
chance to look at ourselves and others as part of the human family, part
of one world. Can we extend this attitude out to the nonhuman world
as well?

I was teaching a retreat in Western Canada recently, not far from a
protest in which several students tied themselves to old-growth trees
being cut down for local paper mills. "How are we to deal with the
complexity of this common situation?" one student asked me. The more
I listened to the competing views, the more I understood the tensions
in the debate. The forestry workers needed to support their families, the

paper mills were looking at the bottom line, and the protesters wanted
to maintain the last untouched forest in the area, never mind what
the fish and rivers had to say. What was most interesting to me in this
situation was that everyone involved, from pulp-mill executives to the
salmon in the forest rivers, lived in the same local community. Since
everyone knew each other on both sides of the debate, nobody could
simply say, "These are awful, nasty people. The planet would be a fine
sort of place if they weren't doing this." The reality, everyone knew, was
that they are doing this and they are people just like us. They are trying
to look after their families and to get ahead in the world. In order to
do anything to protect the forest, we had to find ways to include them.
How do you involve the people who are cutting down the forest? How
do you include the merchants who are paying them? How do you include the civil servants who are taking the bribes to allow the cutting?

According to yoga, duḥkha comes out of people not understanding
how they are creating suffering for themselves and for others. Problems
and suffering come from attachments (rāga) and aversions (dveṣa). You
can't simply wish that away. You've got to work on the basic problems
of bringing knowledge and education into the community. Why were
they cutting down the forest? Of course, they wanted to live comfort-
ably, to look after their families. So, we have to find ways to provide
for them. Otherwise, it would be like trying to build a wall to stop the
tide from coming in. Good luck! It's going to find a way. Instead, you
have to think clearly and find ways to address peoples' needs, to include
them and bring them in. This takes time. You can apply this practice of
honest listening without clinging to views to troubles in your own community, family, body, and mind.

What are all the different causes of the problem? What kind of end
can there be to that problem? If we haven't understood the problem, we
won't be able to see the causes. And if we aren't really clear about the
goal we are working toward, we won't really know what kinds of paths
to develop. It works in society the same way it works in our own practice. The more we reflect on and practice with those truths for ourselves,

the more we are able to apply them in our life, in very ordinary situations, with our friends, with our family, at work, with different problems happening in the community.

The trouble of course is that there are species with no voice. Julia Butterfly Hill, best known for living in a 180-foot-tall, 600-year-old California redwood tree for 738 days to prevent loggers from the Pacific Lumber Company from cutting it down, describes her descent from the canopy of her tree home:

> I climbed into Luna's branches knowing only that it was horribly wrong to turn beautiful forests into clearcuts and mudslides. Seeing this devastation from a treetop perspective raised my awareness and inspired me to act on behalf of all life. In my 738-day vigil I withstood 90 mph winds during two powerful winters, harassment from a helicopter which nearly tore me out of my perch 180 feet high in the tree, and the tremendous sorrow of witnessing the trees surrounding Luna crash to the ground. These were some of the hardest experiences of my life emotionally, mentally, physically and spiritually. Yet I was determined not to let my feet touch the ground until I had done everything in my power to protect Luna and make the world aware of the plight of our ancient forests.[11]

How we speak with each other is the key to relational yoga. Karma operates in the three spheres of body, speech, and mind. When we see that language is an instrument for either hurt or connection, separation or coming together, we see that language is part of the web of life. James Boyd White outlines the domain of language as follows:

> Language, after all, is the repository of the kinds of meaning and relation that make a culture what it is. In it . . . one can find the terms by which the natural world is classified and represented, those by which the social universe is constituted, and those terms

of motive and value by which action is directed and judged. In a
sense we literally are the language that we speak, for the particular culture that makes us a "we"—that defines and connects us,
that differentiates us from others—is enacted and embedded in
our language.[12]

Dialogue is a community-based practice. A self in communication with
others is a personality becoming flexible and open. A workable conception of self, from the perspective of yoga, is that "individuality" comes
to be situated upon the foundations of community, culture, history, and
language. The individual self develops upon this foundation as an in-
heritor of the cultural achievements that have come to fruition in that
tradition. Thus situated, the individual develops a capacity for involve-
ment within the socially structured world. Communication, especially
in difficult times, is simply another aspect of the web of life, always
growing, always changing, always in dialectical relationship.

We need to be able to think big and think small at the same time.
Big ideas require small steps that often begin in the silence of not knowing. From that silence, listening allows new forms to emerge. The quest
for peace and the abolition of war will be long and will require us to dig
deeper into the very depths of the human and institutional psyches that
lead "civilized" peoples to resort to force, and, hopefully, to find and reinforce what is now an elusive culture of peace. Genuine peace requires
the advent of a new selflessness, a willingness to see our fellow humans
as our brothers and sisters and—as the traditional religions have always
counseled—to love them as we love ourselves.

All humans should have the right to a full and satisfying life. For an
individual this means developing his own and his loved ones' potential
growth, and reaching out to his neighbors to help assure that they have
the same chance. For communities, this means developing fair regulations for living together, and encouraging programs that will enhance
fellowship among their many diverse elements. For nations, this means
encouraging their citizens to strive for the enhancement of a benign

attitude toward all elements of their own society and toward all other nations. Peace cannot be oversimplified. Recall that Patañjali uses the term ahimsā, nonharming, rather than śānti, a simpler term that means "peace." There will always be some degree of violence in our actions.

When deciding to protest against their government's actions, the Burmese monks looked at the ways in which they were cooperating with the established government. The monks decided that since the government benefited from supporting the monks through the gift of alms, they would no longer accept alms, and in a strong gesture of non-cooperation, the monks put their alms bowls down.

There is an urgency to this kind of transformation. We are no longer in a technological age or, as many academics would put it, a postindustrial age. Rather we are in a time that calls for understanding complexity and learning how systems work and learning how to work together. In addition to this kind of thinking, we also need to work with our minds. So how can we integrate flexible thinking and listening with ethical action? The answer begins in our mental attitude and our ability to find clarity of mind with less self-referencing. Most of our habitual thoughts are stories about ourselves, and as we learn to work with these habit energies, we learn how to take in situations without filtering our experience through narratives of I, me, and mine.

Rather than thinking of the yamas, then, as a kind of commandment from above, like two stone tablets entrusted to humans by an all-powerful god, the yamas are manifestations of Indra's web, or net. Indra's net symbolizes a universe where infinitely repeated mutual relations exist between all members of the universe. This idea is communicated in the image of the interconnectedness of the universe as seen in the net of the Vedic god Indra, which hangs over his palace on Mount Meru, the axis mundi of Vedic cosmology and mythology. Indra's net has a multifaceted jewel at each vertex, and each jewel is reflected in all of the other jewels. They are reminders of how we can return to the interconnected nature of reality. To return to reality means to let go of the thought patterns that encase, enclose, and frost our ability to see.

Teilhard de Chardin considered this question carefully. "I don't know why, but geologists have considered every concentric layer forming the Earth except one: the layer of human thought. There is no thought but man's thought," he realized[13]—particles spinning, earth turning, thought being modified by further thought. We begin to see that if we can't work with the modifications of thought, we are always at a perceptual distance and disadvantage. How can we take in anything when the mind is stirred and agitated or overconfident and literal? Whether we are looking at sunflowers in rural France or the transparent black of the night sky, layers of thought stand between reality and our version of reality unless we learn how to work with the habitual movements of mind. Without a clear sense of what it is that we are perceiving, thinking, and making choices about, our decisions are based not on reality but on what we hope reality will be.

The more we relax into the present-centered awareness that comes from reducing our habits of reactivity and distraction, the more we find ourselves embedded in a life of life-giving relationships. If we continue to think that our technology or even a transcendent universal god or deity is going to save us from our troubles, sins, or ecological stress, we are fooling ourselves with more stories of mind. Being members of Indra's web, it is our responsibility to take action within the web. We *are* Indra's web.

The industrial world we have created and its products—suburban highways relying on cars, youth transfixed and transfigured by video games, sprawling roads leading to other sprawling roads—cannot be sustained. When the industrial world was created, there was little awareness of its negative side, and now we are living in it.

We are numb to the suffering of the human and nonhuman world because we keep avoiding our suffering through sensual gratification. Opening to suffering is not a negative spiral or a burden in any way at all; rather, human difficulty puts the meaning of our lives into exceptional clarity and context. The more we gratify the senses through transient and artificial means, the more the senses shut down. Eventually we are no longer sure what is good for us. We forget what it feels like to feel and see and hear.

Let us, with compassion, vow to bring to realization humankind's deep desire for freedom and construct a world in which everyone can truly and fully live. In his essay "Nature and the Environment," J. Krishnamurti writes, "Look at the evening star or the new moon without the word, without merely saying how beautiful it is and turning your back on it, attracted by something else, but watch that single star and new delicate moon as though for the first time."[14] If I can feel connection with the moon, stars, and dazzling night sky, a connection so deep I become lost in it and at once completely myself, I can do the same with others; the possibility is always there. Honesty in the context of karma means recognizing the fact that what you do and what happens to you are the same thing, that cause and effect are one, not two.

CHAPTER SEVEN

ASTEYA: NONSTEALING

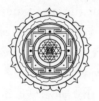

True compassion is more than flinging a coin to
a beggar ... it comes to see that an edifice which
produces beggars needs restructuring.

—MARTIN LUTHER KING JR.

ONE OF THE ways that we can move from viewing yoga as a
social service to a form of social action is to take the core teachings of yoga and employ them as a mode of seeing through the social
and institutionalized forms of duḥkha that we find within and around
us. Offering meditation workshops and āsana classes is the first step
in returning the mind to its natural state, waking up the intelligence
of the body, and bringing more awareness to the ground of reality as
it presents itself in this embodiment. It's important, however, that we
don't reduce the causes of suffering exclusively to the personal realm.
The social fabric that supports greed, hatred, and confusion penetrates
our beliefs and worldviews in so deep a manner that psychologically,
the division between personal and social is a false one.

You and I are each corners of the social fabric, and as such, our practice must include the social sphere and its workings within and around us. A thorough investigation of duḥkha in all its manifestations can't only be personal, because when we work on the personal level, we also work on the social level. Likewise, the two-way-street model should apply to our social and ecological views as well. It's not just that yoga teachings should be put to work on global issues, but that yoga also has much to learn from the excellent social and psychological approaches that many activists have already employed to effect social change and awareness. We must work together. There is no blueprint for the way yoga might tackle global warming or deforestation, suicide or theft. As I've pointed out throughout this book, the yamas are only basic guidelines; how they manifest in the social sphere is going to be a vast and complex challenge for each and every one of us who sees practice as a form of engagement rather than transcendence. When we work to transcend (perhaps "transform" is a more appropriate term here) the habit energies of mind, body, and body politic, we turn *toward* the world, not away from it. In turning toward the social and ecological spheres, we are, in turn, turning toward our own minds and bodies.

Yoga teachings are true only when they are appropriate in given circumstances. Even though I may experience deep stages of meditative samādhi, I still have to get up and buy vegetables, source water, and speak with others. We are never divorced from our social and ecological background, because the background comes through in all of our activities. When we believe that our personal enlightenment is beyond context and outside of any social functioning, we've fallen into a trap. Yoga revolves around the teachings on causality (karma) reminding us that our actions have an effect, that everything we do plants a pattern.

Individual change cannot effect the entire social sphere because it's not a one-way dynamic—the social sphere (and its institutions) are continually informing the individual. Conditioning works in two directions. Though we begin with this mind and this body, we must also

see the way that mind and body are extensions of culture and ecology.
Inner and outer work must happen in parallel if this practice is going to
address global forms of duḥkha.

Practice is consistent with progressive, nonviolent activism, which
occurs everyday when we tend to our families, neighborhoods, and
mind-body balance. I recall the huge inspiration that filled me when
I read Gary Snyder's words on the topic: "The mercy of the West has
been social revolution; the mercy of the East has been individual insight into the basic self/void. We need both."[1] How will yoga serve us
in the long run, so that we create more national parks, less industrial
waste, and yoga practices that revolve around unique community needs
rather than commerce?

Nowhere in the yogic literature do we find specific examples of
community outreach addressing poverty, let alone Internet addiction
or water quality. These are issues of our time, and so we need a yoga of
our time. The core teachings of yoga—including ways of working with
greed and confusion, the selfless nature of "things," and the practices
of settling the mind patterns (citta vrtti)—are essential in beginning
this revolution of the cultural heart. In this way, yoga begins to operate
invisibly through the culture, sticking to the root systems as it makes
its way into the trunks and branches of our unique communities and
families.

Because the ego-self is terrified that it's temporary and ultimately
without ground, it seeks wealth and other external symbols to satisfy
itself, which in turn creates a society structured around such skewed
ideals. Gandhi responds clearly to this kind of illness when he warns
that "there is enough on earth for everybody's need, but not for everyone's greed."[2]

When we take more than we need, we are, in effect, stealing. Of the
five yamas, asteya, not taking what is not freely given, casts the widest
net, especially for those of us embedded in cultures devoted to accumulation and consumerism. What is consumerism? The core notion of
consumerism is that people subject to consumerism overbuy; they pur-

chase goods that they "clearly do not need for subsistence or for traditional display"—more than an objective observer would judge that they
need and perhaps more than they themselves, upon sober reflection,
would admit that they need.[3] But who is going to be the "objective"
observer? People overbuy, according to most descriptions, to emulate
others, to indulge themselves sensually, to escape feeling the reality of
their circumstances, to fill up lack. Consumerism does not refer to basic
subsistence nor to a general life of enjoyment or pleasure but rather
to seeking satisfaction through buying things. This is more than being caught by the sensuality of goods; we are caught in a mythology in
which there is a correlation between duḥkha and consumption whereby
consuming things, we imagine, will overcome or even satisfy our unsatisfied mental states.

We all know what is now a dictum coined by the Rolling Stones,
who wrote, "You can't always get what you want," yet from what we
know about the nature of the mind, we should add that not getting
what you want is not the problem. The problem is that caught up in
fast-paced culture surrounded by goods and advertised needs, you can't
always *know* what you want. Gandhi writes:

> We are not always aware of our real needs, and most of us improp-
> erly multiply our wants and thus, unconsciously, make thieves of
> ourselves. One who follows the observance of Non-stealing will
> bring about a progressive reduction of his own wants. Much of
> the distressing poverty in this world has risen out of the breaches
> of the principle of Non-stealing.[4]

Not stealing means refraining from taking what is not freely given.
This has a broader connotation than nonstealing. The corollaries to not
stealing are generosity, letting go, and contentment. Do we have the capacity to let go? Through opening the doors of generosity, through the
practice of nongreed, we don't create the conditions for harm internally
or externally. Taking what is not given means taking something when

someone is not aware or even cheating someone of something they are not aware of. Exploitation of others or of natural resources also constitutes an act of stealing.

There are people in our practice community who have very little material wealth. They live their lives with great simplicity and follow through with generous promises. I am always inspired by the richness of their lives, and they remind me how little I need to live happily. I feel more comfortable around these friends than I do those who have financial wealth and are constantly troubled by their money. The more we accumulate, the more we have to worry about.

Let's not make thieves of ourselves. Reducing our habits of desire and accumulation goes right to the heart of asteya, nonstealing. Can we do something out of the ordinary and turn our daily desires into new habits of generosity? We are not islands of selves in a sea of people. Not stealing is a way of releasing what is beautiful in ourselves. The vow of nonstealing orients us toward a life free from discontent.

Like a full moon, when the heart is awakened through one's actions, we wake up to bright and buoyant being. The paradox is that even though a moon may sometimes look full and sometimes not, it's always full, only hidden occasionally by shadows. The yamas teach us how to work with those shadows to reveal the brightness of the heart.

Stephen Houseworth writes:

If, in the 1970s, we had asked the question, "What causes crime, what causes people to steal?" most likely people would have said poor parenting causes people to turn out criminal. In the 1980s the fad was that people who committed crime were victims of abuse as children. The 1990s was a time when we heard a lot about the break down of the family unit. Over the past twenty years the assumption was that "something" was wrong with the family. Interestingly, if we go back fifty years we would find the popular theory had to do with poverty and unemployment. Seventy five years ago we assumed the cause had to do with a lack of discipline and, one hundred years ago, the focus was on the lack of morals and religious values. The theories abound and span a list which includes the bad seed theory, peer pressure, the state of the economy, family values, our diet, the effects of fluorescent lights, bad eye sight, learning disabilities, etc. . . . Today researchers are busy looking for the "crime gene." All of these theories subscribe to what is known as the "causal model" of crime. The causal model is one which has an underlying assumption that there is a "cause," something wrong inside or outside of the person which is the source of their criminal behavior and, if this cause can be identified, the person can be cured. The causal model was ostensibly one which was worth pursuing; after all, it served the medical profession quite well. In medicine we can find a germ or bacteria and kill it to make the patient well. In the social sciences this causal model has not proven itself, in spite of 100 years of research.[5]

So what is missing in the causal understanding of theft? Can we see how the root of theft is a reified attention span caught in the belief that taking something will ground me? Any action motivated by craving only leads to more craving. If our desires are endless and if self-image is inherently empty, no thing can ground us anyway. In this respect, taking what is not given freely only serves to reinforce our negative self-image whose substratum is the belief in insufficiency. In a way, habits of perpetual theft offer us a fixed version of the world and of ourselves in which we do not, and cannot have, enough. Untying this internal knot of insufficiency can be a gateway to freedom. For any type of stealing, the antidote is nonattachment, even if this means letting go of an internalized version of oneself.

The acceptance of an interconnectedness that exists among all living things begins by exiting the kind of thinking where the transformation of society is one thing and the transformation of ourselves is another. In yoga neither takes precedence; these two aspects cannot be separated so easily. If interconnectedness is absent in other theoretical paradigms associated with the study of sexual misconduct, greed, crime, or consumerism, we reduce what we study to something artificially linear. Interconnectedness also pushes us to use our imagination because there is no limit to the angles through which we can look. Whether one looks at consensus or other critical theories, the dualistic approaches of "us versus them," "criminal versus noncriminal," "proletariat versus bourgeois," or "man versus woman" all provide fetters that seek to restrain educators, politicians, and good citizens from looking at the reality of our ills. The result is an anthropocentrism that not only exaggerates and misrepresents the importance of the human in the larger scheme of things, but also has the effect of denying what is essential to our being human: our intimate and integral connection to all else.

In *The Republic,* Plato recounts a dialogue between Socrates and Glaucon, Plato's older brother. In it, Glaucon argues that only the fear of detection and punishment prevents a human being from breaking the law and doing evil for the sake of his own self-interest. Glaucon thinks that this natural fact is demonstrated by the shepherd Gyges, who found a gold ring that made him invisible whenever he twisted it on his finger. (According to the story, he found the ring on a corpse in a hollow bronze horse, which was revealed when an earthquake opened up the ground beneath his flock.) On realizing the ring's power, Gyges used it to seduce the queen, murder the king, and take the throne. Glaucon's claim then is that every one of us, however law-abiding and good we might seem, would do as Gyges did if we could avoid detection and punishment. And, Glaucon claims, we would be right to do so, since each human being's only interest is their own self-interest, and we have no interest in justice and morality for their own sakes.

This odd picture of human nature has been accepted by many philosophers since Glaucon, and, indeed, by many other people as well. It raises the following crucial question: When and why should we trust others, if we think that only the fear of detection and punishment prevents them from harming and stealing from us? Glaucon's answer is not enough but touches on something important—the social matrix of human relationships.

We are not, in our study of the yamas, attempting to arrive at some final, transparent, eternal truth that is outside the realm of human choice or human fault. The attempt in this book is to understand the yamas as transhistorical suggestions for transformation individually and culturally and for how one can sustain an ethical, sensitive, and compassionate life. The yamas require no theological commitment, no belief in an afterlife, no creation story or model of a divinity that punishes or rewards. The yamas humanize ethical responsibility by sensitizing us to the intentions behind our actions and the consequences of our actions. To stick to a set of fixed goals and to insist on reaching those goals is often sheer blindness. Shifting our viewpoint is the gestalt shift that is crucial to wisdom, to intimacy, to freedom. The yamas teach us to be alive to the internal relations between all forms of life.

Like all forms of life, human life is relational. When we meditate on our actions, we notice the internal and external effects of our actions. This means that each human being must consider how others behave, and how they will respond to his or her own behavior, in deciding how to act him- or herself. Even Gyges had to do this, in order to achieve dastardly ends. Thus the possibility of relying on each other to behave and respond in predictable, manageable ways is particularly valuable for all of us.

Upon what basis do we make decisions about how we make choices? Should we have objective rules about how we should all behave? Should it be relative and situational? In yoga, ethical decisions have both objective and subjective components. The five yamas are like precepts we practice that straddle the objective (universal vows) and the relative (how they apply in any given context). Sometimes we might articulate the yamas as universal truths, and at other times they are totally dependent on circumstance. This is, however, not a paradox.

When we treat the yamas as objective, it means that when we steal, we transgress a basic natural law of causality causing negative effects in the web of reality. When we lie or kill or steal, we can't commit those acts without unhealthy states of mind. When we act from greed, hatred, or delusion, we set up a chain of cause and effect whether obvious or not. How we condition the mind shapes the culture we live in; our actions set up the condition for future experiences.

The subjective way of looking at the yamas consists of three basic criteria: (1) Are your actions going to cause harm for you? (2) Are your actions going to cause harm to some other being? (3) What is the quality of the intention in the choice you're making?

In terms of the last point, is the characteristic of my intention influenced by greed, hatred, or delusion? When the mind is not distracted and when we are grounded, we can decipher these states of mind more clearly than when we are distracted.

Can we cultivate actions based in the intentions of love, generosity, and benevolence? What is the texture of my intention? In living the yamas as guidelines, we live as though we were consistently present, generous, and attentive. But since most of us are preoccupied and distracted, when we find ourselves about to cross the line and break the yamas, just as a precept is broken, can we stop and look and see what we are doing? The yamas, when treated like precepts, become mirrors in which we can see the web of connections in our mind and habits. And if we follow the precepts blindly, we can fall into self-righteousness, dogmatism, or fundamentalism.

When we set our feet upon this path of cultural awakening, we begin to discover that honesty and nonstealing are essential principles that keep awareness focused on what is important. We are never at a distance from practice, because our everyday activities continually support community. Whatever we observe we change as we observe it, and thus we become filters of society, tied together with everything. Give "this" and "that" a name, and we've already changed it. The universe is always enriched when we are at ease. From this place of ease and nonseparation, we see homeless people on the streets and we see ourselves on the streets; we look into the toxic waterways and we see the river-meridians (nadis) of our own bodies; and we look into collective apathy and we see our own difficulty in knowing what should be done. But we have to do something, and so we begin where we are. We begin with our own body, our close relations, and the food, water, and air supply we all rely on. Our actions become one piece of the whole evolving picture.

Asteya reminds us that yoga is not a practice or viewpoint that is world-denying, but rather one that is life-affirming. Karma can be reformulated so that the old interpretation of karma as bondage to the world can be harnessed in a direction that stimulates intimacy with this very life and moral responsibility for the natural world. Can self-reflection enlarge our capacity to take in others and see ourselves with the matrix of all living systems?

After Patañjali describes the yamas in the second chapter of the *Yoga-Sūtra*, his third chapter outlines the absorption of the human mind in the natural world:

> As one concentrates on the sun, one gains knowledge
>   of the natural world.
> On the moon, knowledge of the ordering of the stars.
> On the polestar, knowledge of their movement.
> On the central energies of the body,
> Ordering of the body in its natural state.[6]

If one of the goals of yoga is to cultivate clearer sense perception, we can see how this moves the practitioner into deeper intimacy with the natural world. The combination of this kind of worldly-responsiveness (without clinging) and increased awareness helps one overcome greed and the consumptive material addictions that are harmful to the ecosphere. Karma reminds us that moral responsibility rests squarely on our shoulders.

CHAPTER EIGHT

BRAHMACARYA: THE WISE USE OF SEXUAL ENERGY

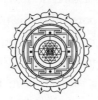

One can ask what might it take to have an agriculture that does not degrade the soils, a fishery that does not deplete the ocean, a forestry that keeps watersheds and ecosystems intact, population policies that respect human sexuality and personality while holding numbers down, and energy policies that do not set off fierce little wars. These are the key questions worth our lifetimes and more.

—GARY SNYDER, *Writers and the War Against Nature*

S EXUAL ENERGY—THAT POWERFUL, mercurial weather pattern causing birth and death, love and destruction, and at bottom, so difficult to describe, define, and live with wisely. Is sexual energy personal? Is sexual energy something to get rid of, explore, act out, treat, condone, or none of the above? Of all the forms of energy that move through human life, why is sexual energy so bound up in personal idiosyncracy, cultural repression, institutional fear, community intolerance, psychological perplexity, yet always present and in creative motion?

Brahmacarya refers to the wise use of energy, particularly sexual energy. It's interesting that Patañjali mentions using sexual energy wisely right at the beginning of his description of the spiritual path. Of course Freud began his description of psychological change in a similar way. When one begins working with the unconscious, whether in mind or body, certain patterns of energy arise that need tending to. We need to learn how to live with and best express hitherto unconscious or imbalanced energies, whether they are sexual, emotional, or purely physical, or combinations and permutations of all these patterns. In the case of sexual energy, perhaps it may be a more difficult energy to work with because there is very little support in our culture for being wise with sexual energy and coming to terms with a true expression of ourselves as sexual beings.

Brahmacarya can be loosely translated as "a code of conduct," "dwelling in Brahma," "a path that leads to Brahma," "moving in Brahma," "abstinence from that which distracts one from Brahma," "the conduct of Brahma." "Brahma" comes from the root "brh," which means to expand, much like the way one conceives of creative energy, the potential of a seed, or the brilliant radiance of the sun. "Brahma" in an Indian context, in its myriad forms, refers to the nature of reality, the absolute basis of nature, culture, personality, organic existence, and all that is perceptible. The term "carya" is derived from the root "car," "to move."

If I am a young gay man exploring my sexual identity in a culture unsure of sexual identity and on a yoga path guided by brahmacarya, how do I live with my emerging sexual energy and sexual identity? If celibacy is not my preferred path, what does sexual exploration look like? Is sexual exploration a valid part of the spiritual path? If so what are the guidelines? If not, how do I work with my emerging sexual curiosities?

Sexuality and sexual energy, both intertwined at a psychological level, present important questions for contemporary practitioners. While the questions mentioned above are only a handful, how do we explore the yama of brahmacarya in a contemporary context, rooted in tradition yet adaptable and alive in contemporary culture? As we've discussed in previous chapters, yoga is only a living tradition when we integrate committed practice with critical intelligence and when we struggle with ancient teachings while remaining open to their effect on our basic assumptions about ourselves and the world in which we are participating. A tradition comes alive as we wrestle with it.

UNFOLDING SEXUAL ENERGY

"Brahmacarya," in its etymological, philosophical, and practical use, refers to the way one uses energy in service not of egoic desire or personal preference but rather in attunement to that which is beyond habit and personal predilection. This is not to posit an impersonal transcendent divinity beyond the human realm, but rather to use our ability to choose actions and work with energy in such a way that we are not reinforcing habits of the ego but rather opening to the moving, eccentric, and raw ground of human being. In the pulse of life itself, energy is always moving. In fact, everything that is perceivable, including the organs of perception themselves, is in a process of constant change. Sexual energy, or any energy for that matter, is moving through a self that is also flowing through phases and changes and is, at bottom, movement itself. Energy is always flowing, and whether that energy is magnetically determined to be "I," "me," or "mine" is a choice we make that leads either to awakening or duḥkha. David Loy writes:

> Can attention retain or gain an awareness of its intrinsic non-dwelling nature, even while engaged in coitus? The normal tendency, of course, involves a future-directed and increasingly urgent focus on the release of orgasm; yet, non-attached, unbound attention is not driven to go anywhere or do anything, because it has nothing to gain or lose in itself. In the urge to-

ward climax, can one become more aware of that which does not change, which does not get better or worse?"[1]

When we treat sexual energy as personal, we turn what is a moving impersonal energy into something permanent. Like water, the softest element, sexual energy is shaped by that which it moves along. If the contours of the self cling to the energy as it begins passing through us, the energy cannot unfold, come alive, and pass away. Instead it takes hold of us and makes us feel caught, taken for a ride, and obscures our ability to act clearly and wisely. Or, we try to repress the energy, pushing it underground for a time, precluding the possibility of opening. Non-attachment means being free from fixation, free from trying to ground ourselves by satisfying immediate, endless, and insatiable desires.

Allowing sexual energy to unfold without repression or entanglement is the task of the yogi. That risk is the essential thing, for it creates in the mind a move toward a more stable sanity. It is much like the risk in making art. We face the blank screen of the arising energy, and we can either move from a place of conservative habit or risk being taken in by what is presenting itself. In her profound book *On Not Being Able to Paint*, Marion Milner draws out the risk of authentic action:

One thing I noticed about certain of my free drawings was that they were somehow bogus and demanded to be torn up as soon as made. They were the kind in which a scribble turned into a recognizable object too soon, as it were; the lines drawn would suggest some object and at once I would develop them to make [them] look like that object. It seemed almost as if, at these moment[s], one could not bear the chaos and uncertainty of what was emerging long enough, as if one had to turn the scribble into some recognizable whole when in fact the thought or mood seeking expression had not reached that stage. And the result was a sense of false certainty, a compulsive and deceptive sanity, a tyrannical victory of the common sense view which always sees objects as objects, but at the cost of something else that was seeking recognition, something more to do with imagination than common sense reality.[2]

Too keen to present a version of reality before it is ready to express itself, impatience is not only inauthentic and fearful, but for Milner, "tyrannical." That tyrannical self-centered project that moves us forward ever too quickly is nothing but a preemptive move to claim permanence in an unfolding movement of energy. We can substitute any form of energy here, whether it is sexual energy, creative energy, or any other. In the spaciousness of awareness, sexual energy is seen to be nothing other than the web of the world, a tapestry moving within a larger tapestry but devoid of self. When self arises, dotting i's and crossing t's too quickly—turning doodles into objects—we miss the invitation to participate in reality and instead participate in a fiction of our own making, one step outside of present circumstances.

If we are constantly distracted and living in quick time, our relationships occur as instant gratification and result only in virtual connection, an uninspired intimacy. If sexual energy is not the domain of yoga, our practice will be fragmented and compartmentalized. Nothing is off limits. What are you committed to? To what and in what do you entrust yourself?

SEXUAL ENERGY AND NONATTACHMENT

If brahmacarya refers to the wise use of energy, particularly sexual, it is a teaching in nonattachment. Not clinging to anything as I, me, or mine allows us to relate to what shows up in awareness with more clarity so that we can develop wisdom in action. Sexual energy is a subtle life force, not a gross bodily function.

Even though sexual energy now may not be as repressed as it was in, say, Freud's Vienna, it is still mirrored in contemporary culture in immature ways.

As yoga practitioners we are not alone in critically engaging traditional teachings on sexuality and sexual energy. Canada's leading Anglican archbishop, Rev. Michael Ingham, is making headlines for claiming that the church has a deeply flawed understanding "of sex that has led to morally groundless objections to masturbation, birth control, abortion and homosexuality." The bishop publicly states, "Christianity as a religion stands in need of a better theology of sexuality, a better understanding of the complex role sexuality plays in our human nature."[3]

We are sexual beings. We are also living at a time when we have a better understanding of homosexuality as a basic and natural orientation among members of the culture, as an example, and our spiritual ideals need to maintain contact with our cultural realizations.

In tantric yoga the human's role in the world has more to do with the creative use of the momentum of energy than consumption. Is there a way that one can move with energy, sexual or otherwise, without consuming or being consumed by it?

"Human sexuality," writes Karen Armstrong in *A Short History of Myth*, "was regarded as essentially the same as the divine force that fructified the earth." A divine force that moves through the world, sometimes creating life and sometimes taking it away, but all the while, sexual energy is thought of as impersonal:

> The harvest was seen as the fruit of a hierogamy, a sacred marriage: the soil was female; the seeds divine semen; and rain the sexual congress of heaven and earth. It was common for men and women to engage in ritual sex when they planted their crops. Their own intercourse, itself a sacred act, would activate the creative energies of the soil, just as the farmer's spade or plough was a sacred phallus that opened the womb of the earth and made it big with seed.[4]

It's not the symbolic nature of the sexual instruments that are important here but the larger vision of a sexual energy moving through life itself, rather than sexual energy as moving because of "me" or into a separate "you." Sexual energy belonging to a "you" and "me" complicates the energies of mind and body by turning experience around the axis of personal possession rather than something entrusted to us. Feeling what moves through the body and thinking with what comes through the mind is a liberated way of seeing and being in the world because there is no clinging to movement, no desire for something external to gratify "me." The changing nature of everything also reminds us that nothing is fixed, there is no unchanging bedrock—my categories of thought, my beliefs, my core values, even my sexuality and sexual identity are in constant and elastic motion.

Insight into the fact that we are interdependent energy fields allows us to see the unique characteristics that make "me" and "you" without confusing those characteristics *as* me and you. The sexual energy that produces a child continues on indefinitely not in some godlike way but rather as a flow of ongoing and diverse conditions. One person receives chiseled cheekbones, another a deformed arm. One child finds in her experience a sharp mind, and another child loses her eyesight. These are our given potentials, characteristics, and capacities, but owning these capacities, like owning sexual energy as a possession, adds nothing to our characters nor to our intimacy. In fact possession is the enemy of intimacy. We already have everything we need; nothing else is necessary. It's important that we find a way to integrate our sexuality with an understanding of karma and ethics.

> The conflict between ethics and sex today is not just a collision between instinctuality and morality, but a struggle to give an instinct its rightful place in our lives, and to recognize in this instinct a power which seeks expression and evidently may not be trifled with.[5]

This passage from Carl Jung's "On Psychic Energy" was written in 1948 while Jung was finding his voice after a falling out with Sigmund

Freud. Jung's groundbreaking paper on psychic energy was an attempt to describe and clarify why he was breaking from Freud's early theories. Jung was attempting to describe the mind-body relation not in Freud's scientific or mechanistic language but rather in terms of energy. For Freud, the sexual drive was the most predominant of the instincts, and Jung disagreed. For Jung there are many instincts, from the need to eat and procreate all the way to the spiritual need for connecting to something larger than oneself. In this essay on psychic energy, Jung first began to describe the basic instincts as energies that continually move toward consciousness.

It was probably no coincidence that Jung was looking into the teachings of yoga in order to find a language better suited to his study than the medical, mechanical, and empirical terms of his time. Jung described the instincts or drives as movements of energy that flowed impersonally through the human being. In moving through the individual they also moved through culture.

Jung felt that the collective morality of turn-of-the-century Victorian Vienna was sexually repressed and that of the contemporary Christian religions was likewise. For Jung, the individual was up against a cultural, institutional, and personal repression and had to completely rethink what sexual energy had to do with spirituality, ethics, and one's own psychological health. If repression was not the answer, what was?

> Every advance in culture is, psychologically, an extension of consciousness, a coming to consciousness that can only take place through discrimination. Therefore an advance always begins with individuation, that is to say with the individual, conscious of his isolation, cutting a new path through hitherto untrodden territory.[6]

Despite the heroic language of Jung's project, we can place the modern yoga practitioner in the same boat: How do we respond to the gaps created between ancient systems of thought, in this case Patañjali's *Yoga-Sūtra,* and contemporary lifestyles, activities, and ethics?

Many times the pursuit of sexual gratification is based on feelings of loneliness or isolation. We want to connect with another—physically, sexually, intimately—as a means of satisfying what we feel is missing or, more positively, expressing ourselves. There is no doubt that intimacy provides satisfaction, but when we split sexual desire from the honest need for intimacy, we end up in a fragmented situation because our sexual expression is split. However, it's important not to create opposite categories where we turn the ego into something "bad" or "wrong," because this will lead to an idealized understanding of spiritual practice. The idiosyncrasies through which our sexual energy moves give us character, and even though we each have various styles and interests, we can still allow sexual energy to move through us without clinging. Like the other yamas, brahmacarya is designed to bring awareness in line with how things actually are, not how we want them to be, and as such, we must cease to think that sexual energy is "I," "me," or "mine," or that sexual identity (and of course any identity for that matter) is fixed. Can we experience sexual energy without forcing our relationships into impossible forms and without using sexual energy as a means of avoiding other aspects of our lives? The feeling of loneliness, as an example, is part of the human condition, but it distorts our human condition when we try to numb loneliness with superficial means. Sometimes it is loneliness that propels us into new horizons as we seek to connect with something more meaningful than our previous patterns.

Brahmacarya, at bottom, has to do with emancipation from self-concern. Can we use sexual energy in a way that gives us access to something greater than our own perspective? It's important that we take the notion of brahmacarya and think through how it might work in relation to our own cultural assumptions and ideas about sexuality, sexually energy, and sexual identity. Sexual energy must always be explored in relation to sexuality and sexual identity in general because it's an energy that moves through us physically, psychologically, and culturally. In early twenty-first-century Western culture, as an example, homoeroticism has become sufficiently open to discussion to be explored publicly, politically, and emotionally, even in the news media, yet it is insufficiently integrated into a general discussion of spirituality to make a worthy topic of sustained spiritual reflection. Topics of sexuality can't be off limits in a practice that teaches us to sit with whatever is occurring with interest and patient curiosity and an investigative stance.

Allen came to our practice center after he spent three months at an ashram, where, in the silence of retreat, he began to feel hatred for himself for always being overwhelmed by sexual energy and not being able to, as he put it, "finally let it go, once and for all, so I can focus more on my spiritual life." He described feeling sexually aroused as soon as he was by himself away from other practitioners and described it as "wanting to masturbate or fantasize or imagine possible scenarios with roommates—but I want all that to go away so I can get this devil out of my skin."

"What about allowing it to be there?" I asked him.

"That would be like an animal caught in a trap," he replied.

"What about leaving the animal alone?" I said.

"I can't rid myself of this. It's always what I most hate about myself and also what I just want to follow. It is a contradiction in me . . . I don't want any more conflict like this."

Allen came to realize that the environment of monastic spiritual practice was bringing some of his distractions to the forefront and some of the compulsion that came up for him when he felt sexual energy was "bad and something to get rid of." But the compulsion itself was the problem, not that it was sexual in nature. Nor was his practice the problem. The awareness was going down into the mind-body depths and touching some very basic patterns in him.

Our work together was to treat sexual energy and his sexual life as sacred and to treat the compulsiveness as the problem. Self-cherishing needs to be neutralized and then transformed into genuine care for others, but when we are caught in self-judgment, doubt, or repressive notions of ourselves, we fix our ways of knowing into impossible corners. The trouble for this young man was living in a contracted and relentless way. What was being trapped was sexual energy, when what should have been caught was the contraction he was creating around the sexual energy, deeming it "bad," "the devil," and "something to be rid of forever." But like any energy or sound or taste or thought, sexual energy is part of our basic humanness. How can we work with the energy in such a way as to respect it and allow it to move through us? How can we create space for the energy to live without repression? Hating ourselves for our compulsions only serves to deepen the compulsive groove.

This practice does not eliminate deeper patterns and habits; it actually brings those very energies to the surface. Even the deep vāsanas (latent impressions), for which we have no perfect explanation of their roots, dispose us to patterns of reactivity that can also be included in the practice. The mind-body process is elastic, not fixed. Under the guidance of a teacher and with the support of community and practice, we can begin to recognize even subtle patterns of brain circuitry laid down through previous actions and ancestry. The more we identify with the past—with what has already occurred—the more difficult it is to change our present circumstances. Through increasing awareness of our predispositions and misconceptions, we can open up space that interrupts the quick reactive impulse of the mind-body habit energies. Since our experience of ourselves relies on the interplay of past memories, associations, and dispositions, undoing the momentum of past habits plays a crucial role in allowing self-image to drop away, even when the energy of habit is powerful, like sexual energy in the case of Allen.

CELIBACY AND MARRIAGE

The trouble with sexual energy is not sexuality per se, but clinging. The deep patterns of attachment (rāga) and aversion (dveṣa) that give rise to duḥkha can be undone by entering fully into sexual energy without clinging. Whether we are in sexual relations with another or not, we can always work with our habits of preference. Sometimes the habits we need to work with are not even personal but cultural. Every culture has values around sexual energy that influence our own preferences and beliefs.

Another area in need of focus is the contradiction in the common assumption in spiritual communities that celibacy and marriage are somehow opposites—one ostensibly involving no sex at all, and the other, again supposedly, involving as much sex as one or both partners might like at any one time. But on reflection, this assumption is also a perplexing cultural fantasy that does not bear close, analytic scrutiny. The generally assumed disjunction between celibacy and marriage is not to be as profound as it seems when we see that sexual activity and sexual energy are not one and the same thing. Rather, the reflective, faithful celibate and the reflective, faithful householder may have more in common—by way of learning how to work with the power of sexual energy—than the unreflective or faithless celibate, or the carelessly happy, or indeed unhappily careless, householder. The point is how we work with sexual energy without unconscious habit energies on the one hand or repression on the other.

Working with celibacy as a precept or vow is certainly not repression. Certainly the rethinking of celibacy and faithful vowed relations (whether heterosexual or homosexual) in an age of instantly commodified desire and massive infidelity is a task of daunting proportions. We can only begin to see that sexual energy can be used wisely when we live it; otherwise we turn this ethical suggestion into a law or an unbreathing statue. Sigmund Freud would agree with Patañjali that sexual energy used wisely provides a means of positive transference of energies. The Christian bishop and saint Gregory of Nyssa, known for his argument that since God is infinite he cannot be comprehended, wrote a wonderful passage on the way in which celibates and married people can be equally involved in a lifelong ascetical exercise. He sounds much like a yogi in chapter 7 of his treatise:

Imagine a stream flowing from a spring and dividing itself off into a number of accidental channels. As long as it proceeds so, it will be useless for any purpose of agriculture, the dissipation of its waters making each particular current small and feeble, and therefore slow. But if one were to mass these wandering and widely dispersed rivulets again into one single channel, he would have a full and collected stream for the supplies which life demands. Just so the human mind . . . , as long as its current spreads itself in all directions over the pleasures of the sense, has no power that is worth the naming of making its way towards the Real Good; but once call it back and collect it upon itself . . . it will find no obstacle in mounting to higher things, and in grasping realities.

When sexual energy is married to wisdom, each and every moment holds no obsessive worry for us. Grounded in stillness, sexual energy becomes just another wind passing through the mind-body process, an impersonal current contingent on conditions that too are contingent on other conditions arising and passing away like all basic constituents of nature. No longer crowded by the constant claims of personal identity, we are free to move *with* sexual energy as a form of true self-expression. Such an expression is the manifestation of samādhi, the experience of integration, an act occurring without a privileged self.

A meditation on sexual energy returns us to the body. Contemplating the energies of the body places us squarely in the hands of nature. "The sun shines not on us," writes John Muir, "but in us. The rivers flow not past, but through us, thrilling, tingling, vibrating every fiber and cell of the substance of our bodies, making them glide and sing."[7] The sun shines through us in the same way sexual energy moves through us. So too they both nourish us and give birth to our very existence. On a path that includes sexual energy as a valid object of meditation, what does a mature practice look like? If sexual identity is not fixed and if sexual energy is as impermanent as any other natural phenomena, can the wise use of sexual energy teach us about the natural world?

It is not *what* we see, yoga reminds us, but *how* we see. Seeing life clearly, what in Sanskrit is referred to as vidya, involves full engagement with what we are seeing and less pushing and pulling of habit. The yamas suggest just the kind of engagement that is required so that we move into ever new affinities with all energies including sexual energy. By tuning in to the places where we are deluded by, caught in, and unskillful with sexual energy, we open up to our basic nature. Then we can get to know sexual energy, on its own terms, teaching us something about the way things actually are.

CHAPTER NINE

APARIGRAHĀ:
NONACQUISITIVENESS

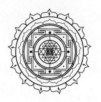

WE ARE NOT concerned to know what goodness is," writes Aristotle in *Nicomachean Ethics*, "but how to become good men, since otherwise our enquiry would be useless."[1] Yoga presents a complete reversal of our perceptual habits and thus a retuning of the world itself. The direction of unlimited desire and egoic satisfaction cannot be sustained any longer. We are pressed at certain points in our lives to reimagine a way of communicating and a means for taking loving action so we don't spin once again through the old turnings of the satifaction-disatisfaction cycle of saṁsāra. Letting go of the ways we accumulate ideas, knowledge, categories, and stories of others is the beginning of inner renunciation. Coming back to the breath, the body, and this moment as it materializes gives us something to abide in other than distracted habit energies. Here is where we take refuge.

In a more extroverted sense, aparigrahā reminds us that nothing actually belongs to us in the first place. In genuine harmony with the natural world we are more concerned with authentic living than with the possession of goods and, sometimes, a relinquishment of such possessions—a voluntary willingness to live with less—is itself a path of authenticity. Even for economically poor people, living simply is possible.

Yet for the truly poor, there is often no choice, which reminds us that choice comes with responsibility. Can aparigrahā remind us that there is more to life than appearance, accumulation, affluence, and marketable achievement? I am reminded of the apocryphal dialogue between an ambitious city person and a Wyoming rancher who was shocked to find the interloper building a cabin on a remote corner of the rancher's vast estate:

Rancher: This is my land, what are you doing here?
City man: I am building a cabin. Who says it is your land?
Rancher: I do.
City man: How did you get the land?
Rancher: My father left it to me.
City man: How did your father get the land?
Rancher: His father left it to him.
City man: And how did your grandfather get the land?
Rancher: He fought the Indians for it.
City man: Fine, I'll fight you for it.[2]

When we enter any kind of relationship, any intimate sharing, renunciation is required. Renunciation is the deep letting go that happens when we decide to meet life as it is, described in the Upanishads as saṁnyāsa, without being caught up in the ambitious desires of the personal and collective ego. Yet renunciation is often misunderstood as leaving behind the world and entering something beyond time and space, outside of culture, and contrary to material progress. This was summed up by Eleanor Roosevelt after her visit to India:

Prime Minister Nehru is trying to develop a democracy that, although perhaps not exactly like ours, will ensure all the people personal freedom. But if an accompanying material prosperity is also to be achieved—and the government will not be successful unless it can demonstrate certain progress on the material side—considerable education and re-education of the people will be necessary. For a belief in the virtue of renunciation is not an incentive to hard work for material gain; but only hard work by all the people is going to bring any real betterment of their living conditions. Somehow a spiritual incentive, a substitute for renunciation, will have to be found . . . My own feeling is that with their religious and cultural background something different will be required to spark in them the conviction that the modern struggle of a highly technologically developed state is worthwhile.[3]

Aside from Eleanor Roosevelt's obvious investment in the virtues and benefits of technological progress, what stands out here is a common misunderstanding of renunciation as isolation or indifference to the world. Of course one of the ways of interpreting renunciation is that leaving the world in an effort to find closer communion with the divine helps one find redemption. Even many interpretations of Patañjali's term "kaivalya" (isolation) hold that the final goal of yoga is ultimate isolation from the world. However, kaivalya refers to the way that awareness stands apart from the changing conditions of phenomena. Though the fluctuations of the mind are always changing, as well as the feelings and thoughts that move through awareness continuously, the awareness itself is unchanging. Awareness is simply aware. Kaivalya describes insight (vicāra) into this separation, not, as many scholars suggest, the yogi's isolation from the world. In fact, through letting go of habitual forms of clinging to thoughts and money and addictions, we find ourselves deeper in the world due to the renunciation of clinging. Renunciation creates the ground upon which we activate our practice.

When we join life—whether through human or nonhuman relationship—we find our true nature, our true home, our refuge. The environmental alienation that characterizes many of our lives separates us from our very ground, the source of life. Gandhi's ethical and religious approach to the treatment of all fellow creatures is founded on an identification with all that lives. His renunciation of ambitious greed became, for him and his followers, a prerequisite to the understanding of profound biological and spiritual interconnectedness, much like the principles advocated by the modern deep ecology movement. For Gandhi the broad ideal of ahimsā, or nonharming, is out of reach unless there is awareness of the interdependence of all of life. And ahimsā was also impossible without self-purification, a largely ascetic life of renunciation of material, psychological, and physical indulgence. Gandhi was an early pioneer of the more-is-less approach to ecologically sound living.

ACCUMULATION IS SOMETIMES subtle. One of the ways we accumulate more than we need is through the mass consumption of knowledge. Accumulating knowledge may produce experts, but experts are not necessarily wise. Wisdom and knowledge do not go hand in hand. In fact one might say that the difference between wisdom and knowledge is flexibility. Unless our knowledge can be flexible and temporarily suspended, even seen through at times, there can be no wisdom.

In our rushed and overscheduled lives, sometimes our pace precludes us from being with the tempo that a body at ease requires. Agitated and used to constant movement, it becomes hard, over time, to rest in psychological stillness, where the mind-body process can receive, assimilate, and respond to life with less reactivity. When the mind is content and the body at ease, even when fully involved in work, our constant desires settle down and the mind can be more discerning when desirous appetite shows up. "Having no real aim," Aristotle astutely observed, "acquisitiveness has no limit."[4]

The problem with accumulation is that it is built on the premise that it will provide some kind of security for us now and for future generations. Hidden in our fantasies of security and permanence is the dazzling reality of our own death and the ultimate impermanence of anything we acquire. At a more existential level, self-image cannot acquire anything at all because, as we've discussed in earlier chapters, it has no real substantive ground. We should begin to relate to the natural world in the same way that we take care of ourselves. As we take care of these solipsistic and exhausting energies of the mind, we begin taking care of the natural world as well. The root causes of the destruction of the natural world have everything to do with our own destructive patterns of action.

Since aparigrahā extends through all of life, we can't continue to accumulate forms of behavior that reinforce greed, hatred, and confusion. Infinite acquisition degrades the earth as well as one another. Nonacquisitiveness helps redirect energies that support personal and collective competitiveness, judgment, and delusion. Keep in mind, however, that since so many spiritual traditions suffer from a glaring discrepancy between ideals and actions, it's important to approach aparigrahā as a practice rather than a philosophical viewpoint. A householder in the *Prithvi Sukta* suggests:

> O Earth who furnishes a bed for all.
> Let what I dig from thee, O Earth, rapidly spring and
>   grow again.
> O Purifier let me not pierce through thy vitals or thy
>   heart.[5]

Where there is the compulsion to accumulate, there is also the deep fear of death. Fixating on objects in the world makes us feel as though we've somehow stabilized the world. This returns us again to Patañjali's distrust of fixed metaphysical explanations of the world that seek permanence and reliability in an otherwise seasonal reality. Feminist writer, teacher, and philosopher Daphne Marlatt, in an interview about her spiritual practice, says:

> [We are facing] an increasing crisis in terms of what we are doing to the environment. We're establishing this horrible hierarchy of wealth that destabilizes and marginalizes whole sections

of the population. It's not just happening here but everywhere. The capitalist accumulation of profit is an economic system that we seem to be stuck with, and it doesn't have a very happy scenario. We can't keep accumulating at the loss of everything else, the precious resources that fuel that drive.[6]

We can no longer resort to the Cartesian notion of a mind here and a body over there and a world separate from them both. Western philosophy has, in many ways, hollowed out the world and sectioned off bits and pieces in a way that has helped give us a sense of autonomy and separation from the all-too-physical world. The current health and balance of the natural world depends on human actions, perceptions, and beliefs. Spiritual practice increases awareness of interdependence and the ecoethical ramifications of belief systems that don't recognize how we are intimately woven into the world. Damage to the biosphere manifests locally in the health of your body and your community. No human being anywhere today can be completely free of residues from human-made toxic chemicals. The environment does not just impact human health; it *is* human health.

The ability not to be enclosed in a given belief system, but to be alive and adaptable in this current moment at this current time in this very body can give us a potent sense of our own capacities and responsibilities. But as we find more freedom in our choices, we also find more responsibility.

Freedom and responsibility go hand in hand, and aparigrahā, the release of acquisitiveness, sharpens our ability to see the effects of our choices individually and collectively. In this interdependent world we need to make choices that best serve the infinite web of interconnections rather than our individual preferences. Intellectually, the term "infinite web" seems looming and philosophical, and obviously it is impossible to predetermine the effect of all of our actions. But we can certainly bring more and more clarity to the kinds of choices we make and to the beliefs that inform those choices so as to maximize the benefits of them for all living and nonliving reality. When we learn to live interdependently, we begin to see that we can enhance the quality of our lives and in doing so also better serve other beings. The quality of others' lives has a direct impact on our well-being; the energy of generosity, as an antidote to acquisitiveness, establishes the reciprocal loop of happiness that occurs when we take others into account while making choices.

Our capacity for destruction of all kinds is also quixotic evidence for our capacity for reconstructing and reimagining this natural biosphere. The same creative energy that we have unleashed against the natural world, as well as one another, can be reoriented and put to use in a way that creatively supports the biodiversity that can put life back on track. Imagine a scientific and technologically imaginative community that is supported by the public to rethink, retool, and rebuild the power plants, toxic industries, and outdated education systems. We wouldn't even need to turn our back on the progress of the past but rather round out our science in such a way that interdependence becomes the primary building block of any new viewpoint or creation.

Ecology is not environmentalism, because it goes beyond the human-oriented perspective and takes into account the integrity and balance of living sentient and nonsentient systems. An ecological viewpoint (the perspective I am attempting to tease out of yoga practice) sees any system as a process rather than a structure. In the same way that the body has immune functions, so too does the earth, as well as the social spheres. We all have the capacity to heal imbalances even though ecological sustainability may take a long time to reestablish itself. Wholeness (samādhi) is not oneness but the dynamic balance of difference among systems. When we can respect and explore difference, intimacy arises.

KARMA AND ECONOMICS

When there is trouble in an economy, the first thing we hear in the news media is that we need more growth. But how much is too much?

Even when growth soars, the benefits are not distributed equally. Furthermore, growth always entails an expansion of industrial production, causing a negative impact to the resources that we call "the natural world." We are at a time now where we've strained every ecological system to the point that the climate is changing and we have no new solutions. Further industrial growth will make life ecologically worse. The yogic alternative to unlimited growth is to see humans as living *within* nature, *as* nature, and not apart from it in any way.

When we see the intimacy of all spheres, no ecologically devastating decision can be economically good. When we imagine nature and human values as separate categories, we end up seeing no moral connection between economies, forests, animals, and waste. What does the natural world become if we only see its value through the lens of the market economy?

Although karma may be a theory of cause and effect, it has no traction without ethical considerations. An example of how causality can be misconstrued by not understanding it in terms of the yamas can best be seen in the work of economist Adam Smith. Adam Smith is one of the creators of the contemporary capitalist system of economic activity that dominates the global markets and influences in drastic and subtle ways the way we think about economic relationships of all kinds. Smith laid the intellectual foundation that explained the free market and still holds true today. He is most often recognized for the expression "the invisible hand," which he used to demonstrate how self-interest guides the most efficient use of resources in a nation's economy, with public welfare arriving as a by-product. To underscore his laissez-faire convictions, Smith argued that state and personal efforts to promote social good are ineffectual compared to unbridled market forces. He was most famous for dictums such as "Virtue is more to be feared than vice, because its excesses are not subject to the regulation of conscience."

At first this sounds like a good understanding of karma. But let's look a little further. Smith felt that there was an invisible hand at work that transformed the accumulated benefit of self-interest into a greater social good (to say nothing of the environment). "It is not from the benevolence of the butcher, the brewer or the baker, that we expect our dinner," he wrote, "but from their regard to their own interest." An individual acting from self-interest he argued, would be motivated and led by "an invisible hand" that would transfer the benefit of their actions straight into the wider social sphere to the benefit of others.[7] Smith exemplifies what free market advocates argue in their appeal to consumers to buy and to producers to keep on producing. Anything that gets in the way is considered an obstruction to the natural gears of the free market system. But the free market system is not completely free.

ECONOMIC WEBS

Human and all other organisms are members of the system we call planet earth. As members of this system we form a web, knotted together almost invisibly at times but nevertheless intimately and inextricably. We are born from the earth, supported by the earth, and return to the earth, and we need the earth to live. Similarly we need the table of elements and, arguably, each other. The earth is not just what supports us; it's what sustains us. It cannot be considered a commodity, because it is our greatest resource.

If I continually take water from the lake out of my own economic self-interest, I could argue that I'm benefiting others by supplying them with water. But the gears of Smith's machine don't account for the effect of water drainage on the lake nor the effect of my livelihood on relationships between parts of a whole greater than the human whole. Why should humans have the privileged position of determining the effects of self-interest? Certainly Smith's argument has become a form of self-interest compounded by self-interest. But what limits my self-interest? Where do we draw the line?

The free market places a high value on mastering production to meet consumption and then influencing consumption to affect production. The argument for this position is not only that the economy "takes care of things" but that having people employed is the number one priority. If people have money, they can keep the machine rolling on.

Unfortunately it's not working. One of the truths that we have not adequately faced is the fact that capitalism today has become a society, not only an economy.[8] The point here is not to create an economic critique of capitalism but to lay the foundation for understanding the psychology of unrestrained economic models and how that affects us personally and collectively. Our society is made up of individuals making choices, and we need to get down deep into the nature of a mind that is delusively split, fragmented into a me that operates continually out of self-interest with dissatisfaction and unfulfilled desires as a result. How much is enough? Free markets are collective agreements that are not without limitations. Most significant among these limitations is the fact that there is a striking absence of any moral principle governing the distribution of what the economy produces. Even when the economy is doing well, income inequality in industrialized countries tends to increase.[9]

What moves this cycle personally and institutionally is the root cause, duḥkha, namely: greed, hatred, and delusion.[10] Nowhere in the natural world can we find the kind of blind self-interest that we find in the current Western economic model. Although this book is not a study in economics, but rather a study in psychology, economics provides a clear illustration of a culture that is not only split, but does not yet have a means for its people to understand their own minds and the effects of their actions. Everything has to move somewhere.

Can we see ranking systems among animals in the natural world? Yes. Individual acts of aggression and domination by the strongest in animal groups? Yes. But not the institutionalized and immutable system of hierarchy that develops in human societies. Not the relentless energies of greed, ill will, and delusion. In the second instance, the fragility of the world ecology—in other words, of the world's ecosystem— brought almost to its knees by unrestrained habits of desire, reminds us that humans have created a machine that is out of control mainly because it has no internal restraint system. Nothing stops us. The people closest to the effects of our actions—mental-health workers, ecologists, doctors, nurses, teachers, scientists—keep telling us that our very survival depends on the immediate transcendence of our unrestrained lifestyles and shopping habits.

If spirituality is the domain for understanding our place in the world, it is certainly the domain for change. But are we thinking in these terms? Can personal and collective change as a spiritual path offer us valid answers? What is ecology but an understanding of relationship?

Returning to the dialogue about global warming, free trade, poverty, abuse, and other global ills, there should be a reworking of every social structure within the present society to accord with laws of a nonhierarchical nature. Crucially though, this reworking must come from human society—the only repository of reflective ethics—and involve the active imposition of human values on the natural world. In other words, it's not that other animals don't have innate ethical understanding; that would be naive. It's that as humans doing so much damage we need to use our capacity to reflect on the damage done by our competitive (or, me first, top down) approach to the environment in which we live, so that we begin to better the quality of our relationship to the earth, to each other, and to ourselves. This attitude can only be established through pausing, looking, listening, and returning to our senses. We can learn a great deal from the natural world, but only if we can be quiet and attentive. In this way our beliefs are always open to correction, open to change, in time with the flowing syncopation of all things.

What yoga teaches us about our current personal, collective, and ecological ills is that the problem begins with perception. If we could replace our idea of the "autonomous individual" serving his or her "self-interest," we could alter significantly our ideas about progress. Progress in terms of relationship means that we have to monitor our actions so that they become dialectic, always moving back and forth among the web of relations that sustain, support, and ultimately are who we are. What is conducive and sustainable in terms of relationship? Is what

I do good for the earth? Good for the air? Good for my body? Then we can go further: What is my body without earth? Can I even have a body without air? Is there an "I" there at all?

Suddenly we are back in the domain of spirituality. Learning to perceive our lives as situated in the greater whole of organic life—arising, unfolding, and passing away—keeps us connected to the living and breathing whole of which we are made. In yoga nothing can be disconnected. The goal of yoga is vidya—seeing things as they are, being with life as it is, not as we need it to be or expect it to be. Yoga dismantles our basic mode of self-interest, or in more psychological terms, self-cherishing. Yoga teaches us to perceive the world more truly than our habits first suggest. Yoga teacher Esther Myers once told me that what she feels she is teaching within each and every yoga pose is a life of values. "What we give value," she said, "determines the kind of families and friendships we all have. Our values all determine how we relate to ourselves. So the yoga teacher, in how she tells us how to work with the body, constantly instills values of patience and clarity in all of her students."[11]

The yamas are concerned with the values that we live by and the effects of choices we make based on those values. The values are not written in stone, not handed to us through the word of a god, nor are they ultimate laws enforced by a divine judge. Ethics are values that we agree to live by. Understanding the inherent insubstantiality of material things is called "mithyā dṛṣṭi." The yamas, as ethical values, challenge my personal desires and preferences and therefore challenge my egoic ambitions. Turning toward the world without the intent to harm or to accumulate more than I need begins a path of practice whose goal is freedom from discontent and lack. Do you have everything you need to practice?

In a way the Yoga of Patañjali is groundbreaking in that it requires no belief in a metaphysical self but rather an awakening to the inherent insubstantiality of self-image. If we reify Patañjali's teaching as a set of rules or even a fixed theology, we lose what is radical about his or her teaching. The self is seen to be radically linguistic and historical, and such insight not only alters our perception but our moral responses too. A belief in a prefabricated enlightenment is harmful. If we see the spiritual path as a developmental ladder with a pinnacle that is as of now hidden, we continue looking around and outside of ourselves for some vital knowledge that will bring happiness. I am always poking at our students to become fellow travelers and to remember that there are no ready-made truths waiting for a specially authorized person to reveal them to you. Make a friend of not knowing. Open to the body, open to the breath, open to states of mind one after the other, and slowly, tune in to awareness of this very moment free from any theological commitments and free to respond to what is happening. Since we always have only our own eyes and our own point of view, we carry a responsibility to clarify our means of seeing. There is no truth apart from the world. Whether you believe in life after death or an immortal soul is useless when measured against the possibility of tending to what is here right now. And the more we tend to what we are made of, the clearer our responsibility to take care of it becomes. Nature does not have to be something written by god but rather something we are in every sense. There is a wonderful Quaker pamphlet whose title sums it up quite clearly: *There Is Another World but It Is This One.*[12]

Too often we have come to equate life's meaning with the possession of material goods and the pursuit of wealth. The advertisements on television tell us that "success" in life is to have a pleasant appearance, to have money, and to be economically productive. And yet most of us know that there are many forms of work that are just as important as making money. Taking care of parents is a form of success; being a good parent is a form of success; simply being kind to others is a form of success. These deeper forms of success are too often forgotten in consumer culture, and the effects on families and communities have been disastrous. Consumerism and greed have led many people to find more value in life in material things than, for example, in friendship and family and community. We don't have to continue in this momentum. The past nourishes or constrains us; the future calls us. We humans are indeed historical beings, but history does not simply mean the past; it also means the future; and every action we undertake in the present is an actualization of that future. Can we enjoy some consumer comforts without lapsing into greed? Can we become not just economic leaders but moral leaders? Can we be servants of servants?

The yamas, beginning of course with the teaching of nonviolence, assume from the outset that humanity's greatest wish is to not be harmed. I do not want to be harmed by someone else's actions of body, speech, or mind. This is the interpersonal approach to choice and values. Most ethical ideas fall into the domain of not causing harm to other humans.

In terms of the yamas, morality is conceived as responsibility to others, as opposed to the conception of morality as obedience to moral rules. When we stretch the teachings of ahimsā by casting our actions out to a wider range, we come to see that we have obligations to all beings. Aparigrahā applies far beyond the realm of human interaction with other humans and also beyond humans and their interactions with animals. We must include in the net of aparigrahā our actions in every part of every web of life, leaving no stone unturned. Without restraint our perspective too easily lapses into anthropocentrism. One of the most detrimental aspects of Western modernity has been its neglect of the natural world. Shaped by the idea that humans are not part of nature, the West developed in ways that reduced economic development to development for humans, without remembering that human economies are always nested within the larger context of the earth itself.

The yamas are a set of commitments or choices that are expressions of our deep caring, which is our fundamental and inescapable relationship with the world and our place in it. It is because we are at bottom both a "self-project" and a "caring about others project" (that is, we exist as beings who create themselves in time and who must relate in some way to the world outside ourselves) that we must have moral commitments. And to push it one ironic step further, this makes us selves contingent upon a world that is *not* other than this very self. The yamas help us determine what we should be committed to in order to consistently return to our place in the great web of life.

When we watch a building being constructed with no regard for its place in a community, on the street, in relation to the architecture surrounding it, or even its ecological impact, nonacquisitiveness should be a valid method for bringing into question what we witness. If we need this building, how and where does it belong? When we say, "I don't agree with that kind of building," or, "Why are they wasting all this money on such an ugly stadium?" or, "That kind of building is not aesthetically pleasing," we are trying to put words to a sense of discord that has ethical implications beyond the aesthetic. "I think we do this," writes ethicist and ecologist Warwick Fox, "because we don't know how to say in ethically weighted terms what we really want to be able to say."[13]

"When I practice like this day in and day out," says a young woman during a weeklong retreat, "I realize this is no retreat at all. I've been retreating up until now. It is dawning on me that ethics is just something you are, something that does not hold my tongue back when there is something to say. When I'm quiet like this, it's so clear to me what actions of mine are beneficial and what actions just cause trouble."

BECAUSE CONTEMPORARY YOGA in the West does not always occur in organized communities like ashrams or temples, we may not always recognize the importance of restraint and morality in the cultivation of our practice. When practitioners live together or, at least, depend on one another, morality becomes a central issue. It's helpful to see the yamas as personal resolutions that you undertake to help the community as a whole, especially if you see that certain behaviors of yours are creating discord in the community. So in a social sense, the yamas favor community practice. Drinking alcohol, for example, may not be intrinsically harmful, but when we see that our drunkenness decreases our sensitivity to others, we may decide to stop drinking for the sake of the whole. Living in a singular and isolated way, being cut off from community, you may not notice the effect of your alcohol consumption with the same clarity or resolve. Therefore, the yamas can be considered suggestions for social behavior, not as a value system but as a mirror for practice or even a form of devotion to others' well-being. It will never be profitable to strip-mine a mountain. Erosion beyond the balance of soil regeneration is not sustainable intimacy. If we only see nature in terms of accumulation and the marketplace, the natural world becomes nothing but an assemblage of bits and pieces. Taking care of the other, taking care of the earth, taking care of this water supply, is taking care of myself.

CHAPTER TEN

NOTHING IS HIDDEN!

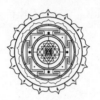

The self is only a shadow cast in grammar.

—LUDWIG WITTGENSTEIN

D URING A CRISIS of faith in which I did not understand the purpose of practice, I asked one of my teachers what this practice was heading toward. "To tell the truth," she said, "I'm really not sure." Just as she finished her sentence, the sound of a woodpecker echoed through the room. I wasn't listening because I was so caught up in my worry about practice and what she might think of me as I was questioning what I was doing. I was worried. I looked up at my teacher and she was smiling, listening to the sound of the bird and studying the light shifting among the dried plants along the windowsill. She was at ease and open, less caught up in the distracted needs of the mind and totally immersed in the play of light and sound in her small and perfect loft space. She looked back at me and a wide smile filled me instantly. "Practice isn't going anywhere," she said. "It's not divorced from anything."

It's interesting how the divorce that splits the world up into "me" and "not me" happens so quickly but also so unconsciously. When I look for what I call "me," all I find is a commentator or rather a commentary without a center. Everything I think of as "me" is a kind of momentum in grammar.

Sometimes we treat our yoga practices grimly, as though there is some place at which we will finally arrive, where the commentary will end and enlightenment will be achieved. Meanwhile the birds are enjoying their pecking, and chirping and the plants on the windowsill are turning toward the sun. What a challenge! The plants are smiling, and the birds don't seem worried.

THOUGH HE TAUGHT many practices, Patañjali is best known for his description of an eight-limbed path known as aṣṭāṅga yoga. Eight limbs are necessary, according to Patañjali's logic, so that our practice leaves no aspect of our life untouched. We move forward in our practice by leaving nothing out until practice and everyday life become one. How can the spiritual and the everyday be considered separate? Where could we possibly draw the line? If any one spiritual path is going to stand the test of time, it must contain multiple paths and techniques to accommodate our idiosyncrasies and also the maturation of our lives. Every system has a shadow once it becomes codified as "a system," so, over time, the path evolves and twists, which is precisely why there are many systems of spiritual practice. Richard Freeman describes Patañjali's system as follows:

> Aṣṭāṅga means "eight-limbs" and refers to a yoga practice, which is evolving into deep, spontaneous meditation and complete liberation. The variety of limbs guarantees that the awareness operates in all spheres of one's life, so that no distortion, perversion or fantasy will attempt to usurp the real yogic insight. In many of the Upanishads the eight limbs are further expanded to fifteen. The advantage of considering the path of yoga to have many aspects is that one is encouraged not to neglect the moral, the ethical, the interpersonal, the physiological, the esoteric and the

meditative aspects of practice. The term Aṣṭāṅga implies both a simultaneous realization of all these interrelated aspects of practice and a logical step-by-step progression where one limb prepares one to truly practice the next.[1]

Patañjali describes in definite and lucid terms the factors of volitional action that help our progress on the path of awakening. Awakening is an accurate way of describing the spiritual path as it captures the concentric process of waking up from veils of habit and delusion. At the same time, we must remember that awakening is not dependent on a path, or anything else for that matter.[2] Pure awareness is unconditioned. Abstinence from dishonesty, falsehood, slander, or any other form of harmful speech is an example of the link between our actions and psychological and social change. The yogi who is honest in action and speech creates a life of clarity in relationship and authenticity in one's self and contributes to an environment with these same qualities.

Abstinence from the taking of life, from stealing, from greed, and from sexual misconduct keeps us from inflicting harm on other living beings and promotes a sense of affinity with other participants in the greater web of life—an expression of our interdependence. When adopted as guidelines to action, the yamas stimulate the growth of healthy mental attitudes and physical well-being that come to expression in ecologically beneficial courses of conduct. The yamas curtail the tide of competition, greed, envy, exploitation, grasping, violence, and war. In their psychological dimension they promote mental harmony, in their social dimension they promote peace, and in their spiritual dimension they serve as the irreplaceable foundation for all higher progress in more subtle states of meditative stillness. Put into ongoing practice, the yamas reverse mental states rooted in greed, anger, or delusion and promote actions rooted in generosity, love, and wisdom, making every situation a portal for awakening.

In our small community of practitioners in Toronto, we encourage each other by taking part in outreach programs that range from teaching meditation and yoga postures to all walks of life, offering support to women making choices around abortion, training clinicians in the integration of contemplative practices in their professional work, and various other ways of bringing these practices into the community. The result of being involved in these projects allows us to continue to bring the insights from practice into the world. For some, these activities are geared toward raising families, and for others, perhaps making music or going for long walks on the lakeshore become expressions of yoga.

When applied toward the continual force of volitional action, the yamas extend our yoga practice in daily life in innumerable ways. In the context of āsana, prāṇāyāma, and meditation, they support the rooting out of harmful energies that distract the mind and create obstacles to meditative awareness. Actions based on nonharming, honesty, nonstealing, the wise use of energy, and nonacquisitiveness are tangible expressions of a corresponding mental attitude. The yamas make our spiritual practice accessible and down-to-earth, rolling our daily life into our spiritual path over and over again. The inner acceptance of ourselves and others begins with a life molded by ethical concerns and commitment to contemplation and action. What is true self-expression?

EXPRESSING PRACTICE

Our actions almost always correspond to dispositions of mind. When I am impatient, traffic moves too slowly; when I am angry, others are irritating; when consumed and preoccupied with myself, other people only get in the way. Patañjali uses the yamas to describe how we can participate in the world and cultivate a spiritual practice with one's body, speech, and mind. This means that we don't need to wait around for the culture to change—the imbalances right in front of our eyes are freshly stretched canvases.

Since volitional action is present in pretty much every state of consciousness, it acquires a distinctive ethical quality when the mind is less reactive and more in tune with the body and present conditions. A highly reactive mind, a body irritated, and a nervous system highly strung is a recipe for unreflective action. Unwholesome choices (akusala) arise from similar mental states, and wholesome actions (kusala) depend on wholesome states of mind. Our mental and physical well-being is the root (mula) of our perception of and activity within the wider world.

The absence of negative mental and physical states signifies not just quietness of reactivity in consciousness, but the presence of generosity, sensitivity, and attunement. Our habits are not irreversible. Past patterns are always malleable and they can be redirected based on the yamas. Actions based on the yamas perfume the mental stream with the qualities for which they stand.

In meditative practice, when the mind becomes still without adding anything to experience and without trying to escape from that particular moment, there is a still and lucid clarity that is nothing other than pure awareness. Without any duality and not depending on anything for its existence, there is naked awareness with no sense of a "me" having the experience. This is the flow of humanness, where, even momentarily, we wake up to what is real and true in a given moment, by means of stillness. This kind of awareness is like a natural resource that is always there, innately stable behind the scenes.

It's hard to resist naming awareness because we want to give words to the experience of nonduality, yet as soon as we do, we enclose the experience. When there is pure awareness, there is no "me," yet "I" am completely there. As you read these words, you can look in your subjective experience for the actual subject who is reading, but you will find that it's hard to locate any trace of "me." The skylarking mind, with its infinite reserve of imagination and distraction, always tries to find a final reference point for each and every moment (kṣana) of experience.

If you look into the sensations in your body, or within the thoughts passing through awareness, or even at your hands flipping pages, you will hardly find the actual location of yourself. That's because the self is a notion, a fiction, and an ongoing construction created conceptually, not ontologically. We are made of 12 billion years of evolution, and this body is the ancestral residue of family and culture and environment. Even the mineral ancestry that makes the human body a living organism can in no way be separated from what I claim to be "me." If I took the nonhuman elements out of the human body, there would be nothing left.

When we see that self-image is empty of basic substantiality, we are sent back into pure awareness, the sense of observing without identifying with ourselves as observers. This experience has been at the heart of mystical traditions for the length of human history. That everything perceivable exists in front of pure awareness and that awareness itself has no distinct shape or form points to the inherent union of the human reality. We *are* nature. If we do not layer concepts on top of our mystical experiences, and if we can allow such experiences to penetrate the way we do our daily lives, and if we no longer associate the "mystical" with anything outside of that on which we rest our attention at this very moment, we begin to see the deep interconnectedness of all life. We see that spiritual is not supernatural, for nothing is hidden, nothing is secretly lurking behind the tree or the river or the mind. This is it!

The freedom to be at ease in the world rests on recognizing the world as being free unto itself and especially free of our idea that the spiritual is a realm separated off from everything of which we are aware at this moment. Do you think there is something else? Do you think yoga practice or any spiritual practice is going to take you away somewhere? What kind of belief system is operating behind the scenes if we think that "the spiritual" is anything other than this? Meditative states of dhyāna and samādhi are not just characterized by concentration but also by the sense that everything is united. Pay attention, this is all there is.

When I don't pull back into my conceptual enclosures, when I allow myself to dissolve in the freedom of pure awareness, I find myself completely myself, which in essence is the freedom to be nobody. This does not mean I am passive. Certainly anyone paddling on the tenth day of a canoe trip or falling deeply through the headphones of a favorite piece of music has experienced the temporary interruption of self-centered perception, only to reveal an awareness free of self.

In the unperturbed present, we notice that it's not awareness that fluctuates, it's the parade of concepts that do. Consciousness that goes after things conceptually is not what we mean by pure awareness. Awareness is always free—that's why Patañjali is so careful about naming it. As soon as we wrap language around awareness, we solidify and conceptualize a mode of seeing and being that is utterly free of such proliferations. Furthermore, awareness is not something we strive to enhance or create; rather, it's the ease that's left when clinging is relinquished.

"Yoga is the release of the fluctuations of consciousness," Patañjali claims in his definition of yoga.[3] He calls the fluctuating patterns of mental distraction "citta vrtti." It is not that we get rid of the turnings of thought and imagination; it's that when we see the citta vrtti, the fluctuations of mind, simply as fluctuations coming and going, we see clearly through them, no longer ensnared by our thought process, but able to notice thoughts and remain centered and responsive in present experience. When we see the fluctuations of mind as reactions to present circumstance, and when we leave such activity alone, present experience bursts forth unmodified. When we see the inherent difference between citta vrtti (the fluctuations of consciousness) and puruṣa (pure awareness), we begin to cultivate the ability to notice our experience from a place of stillness. Patañjali is as straightforward as always when announcing the process of stilling distractions: "Then pure awareness can abide in its very nature."

If the mind is unstable and wavering, we go after every thought, cling to sensations, conceptualize about what we are feeling and experiencing. But pure awareness does not move. The purpose of meditation, breathing practice, and yoga postures is to wake up the mind and body and then allow them to rest in stillness. When the mind is settled and the body grounded and intelligent, we can see life clearly and more simply. When we open joints in the body that were previously glued together, when we spread the breath into stagnating pools within the body, when we learn how to concentrate the mind, our perceptual faculties become clear and flexible.

The yoga postures open the stagnant energies of the body through realigning the energetic pathways of the breath and nervous system. Over time we find that the breath has an astonishing richness as complex as any biosphere with its interweaving strands of birth and decay, transformation and stillness, death and rebirth. As the breath rises and falls, so too does the mind, and we come to see that the natural ecology of mind, breath, and body are indivisible. Mental patterns are created out of sensations in the body, and then our mental attitudes in turn affect those same sensations and give rise to new patterns as well. This seamless and ongoing process moves forward on the fulcrum of the breath cycle as the inhale arises, unfolds, pauses, and then, in turn, becomes the complementary exhale pattern.

All movement is derived from and returns to stillness. The quiet breathing body folded over itself in a forward bend is an expression of both stillness and movement. When we look deeply into stillness, we find subtle movement, and as we find more and more grace in the movements of body and mind, we begin to see how they are expressions of stillness. Don't think stillness and movement are complementary opposites. When we relax into time, when mind and body are synchronized with breathing, there is action with nobody coming or going and the self-created shackles drop away. The quiet mind becomes the marvelous dynamism of the universe, and just like trees expressing themselves in each season, we become who we truly are, and we are home.

When we find meditative stillness, the insight arises that we are evanescent beings, coming and going, being born and passing away. All thoughts, feelings, and everything in our range of perceptions is coming and going. It is through this calming of cerebral activity that we begin to realize an intimacy with all things, which is so thorough it renders all distinctions and concepts simply ideas in the mind. We begin to realize that nothing separates who we are as unique beings from everything that comes to be. Each tree is unique; each bird has specific distinctions; and each human life ages within particular parameters. Our dispositions influence everything that occurs through us. Nothing exists independently of our being and our actions. By splitting away from the basic operation of the world, we create a root schism out of which the separateness of "you" and "I" is born.

Yoga is not a move toward an idealistic belief system of nonduality but rather a guideline for allowing the inherent unity of reality to burst forth into our lives. Rather than thinking of spirituality as a belief in something beyond this world, yoga reminds us that we are no other than this very world as it unfolds in this very moment, beyond any framework of belief. This occurs as we find stillness in mind, life in the body, clarity in relationship so as to recognize that we are a single family, a single body of interpenetrating life-forms. This is not intellectual conceptualization but a move toward conducting ourselves as "one" and relinquishing the what's-in-it-for-me reference point. The distinction between "me" and "nature" or "nature" and "society" seems so fundamental and familiar that it's almost beyond question. Collectively, this ingrains the distinction that not only organizes the imagination and perception of society, but also organizes policy and law. Yoga reminds us that "nature" and "natural" are human-constructed categories. These dualistic designations are cultural-linguistic products freighted with numerous biases, assumptions, and prejudices. Yoga reminds us of the incoherence of such an attitude, and the teachings of karma help us see the consequences of this dualistic view.

Unconsciousness breeds habits, and those habits can also reinforce our ignorance. As Bill McKibben points out, it's even impossible to "get back to nature" because "nature" and "society" were never separated to begin with.[4] The natural and the social are not ontologically distinct. An industrial-led movement has increasingly reinforced this perceptual bias even down to the atomic level where humans can split and genetically modify so-called other organisms, essentially reconstituting nature for our own benefit. However, we have the capacity to reimagine the human, social, and natural worlds in a way that is not dichotomous.[5] We can't just think beyond these dualisms, but rather we must be deeply and viscerally aware of the inherent nonduality of these intellectual and cultural categories.

This state of affairs requires that we move deeper and deeper into our practice so that we can penetrate the levels of mind that set up these conditions in the first place. Maybe you are not an activist in the popular sense of the term, but stillness is a profound form of social action in that it aims to accept, investigate, and transform the roots of our negative habits. It's not that we try to act compassionately or nonverbally, for we are not actors; instead we *become* nonviolence; we *are* compassion.

WE CANNOT SPEAK of yoga independently from its expression in each and every one of us. Yoga itself is the conduct of a person who moves with and of the world, resisting nothing through pure acceptance and acting swiftly out of the recognition that we are one family. A tiger is poached, a child is abused, a window is smashed, and each situation happens to this one body. Yoga is not beyond this body, but rather it is the recognition of union *through* this body, this mind, and this very experience right now; any further conceptualizing limits our ability to respond to present experience here and now. "The whole world," says Śaṅkarcarya in his commentary on the *Yoga-Sūtra*, "is upheld by mutual cooperation."[6] The car outside is idling and I walk toward the driver and, with clear intention, point to our son playing with his tractor next to the exhaust pipe. He turns the motor off.

A mother across the road dresses her daughter in blue and yellow pants, an executive gets in her car, new graffiti appears on the neighbor's telephone pole, and our son's rosy cheeks have been scratched by the cat again. Everything coexists in the big city, a subuniverse of reality assembled together in moving horizons of time.[7] The flower blooms, and the garbage truck arrives.

CHAPTER ELEVEN

JEWELS SHOWER DOWN

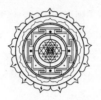

Patañjali's philosophical perspective has, far too often, been looked upon as excessively "spiritual" or isolation-istic to the point of being a world-denying philosophy, indifferent to moral endeavor, neglecting the world of nature and culture, and overlooking the highest potentials for human reality, vitality, and creativity. Contrary to the arguments by many scholars, which associate Patañjali's yoga exclusively with extreme asceticism, mortification, denial, and the renunciation and abandonment of "material existence" (*prakṛti*) in favour of an elevated and isolated "spiritual state" (*puruṣa*) or disembodied state of spiritual liberation, I suggest that Patañjali's yoga can be seen as a responsible engagement, in various ways, of "spirit" (*puruṣa* = intrinsic identity as Self, pure consciousness) and "matter" (*prakṛti* = the source of psychophysical being, which includes mind, body, nature) resulting in a highly developed, transformed, and participatory human nature

and identity, an integrated and embodied state of liberated self hood.[1]

—IAN WHICHER, *"Ethics of Liberation in Patañjali's Yoga"*

I N   T H E   S A M E   way that a word in a sentence has meaning only
in the context of the sentence, or the way a color looks different
depending on the light and other colors in its proximity, humans beings are always grounded in context. Scholar Ian Whicher describes the
clarifying vision of yoga as a practice of action:

> Far from being exclusively a subjectively oriented and introverted
> path of withdrawal from life, classical yoga acknowledges the in-
> trinsic value of "support" and "sustenance" and the interdepen-
> dence of all living (embodied) entities, thus upholding organic
> continuity, balance, and integration with the natural and social
> world . . . Through yoga one gains proper access to the world
> and is therefore established in right relationship to the world. Far
> from being denied or renounced, the world, for the yogin, has
> become transformed, properly engaged.[2]

Human beings need to recognize their function and role within the
larger ecosystem in order to fine-tune their actions so that they have
positive consequences. It's not just that actions determine results but
that our intentions influence our actions. Even deeper still, our belief
systems influence our intentions, and deeper still, we see that our self-
image determines our belief systems. The way I think of my self determines the kind of ideas I have about the world, because there is no
"objective" world "out there" but rather my experience of it as influenced
by my beliefs. Therefore, we must recognize what our basic beliefs are
and how self-image transpires to create "my world."

This ecopsychological perspective places us squarely in and of the world because we begin to see that if we have ideas of ourselves as inherently separate from the natural world and each other, our actions will follow this dualistic mode of perception. We need to maintain the health and integrity of personal, regional, global, and cosmological ecologies. Patañjali suggests:

> The ethical principles are nonviolence, truthfulness, abjuration of stealing, wise use of sexual energy, and absence of greed.
>
> These universal ethical principles, unrestricted by conditions of birth, place, time, or circumstance, comprise the great vow of yoga.
>
> When one is plagued by ideas that pervert these ethical principles and observances, one can counter them by cultivating the opposite.
>
> Cultivating the opposite is realizing that polluted ideas, such as the idea of violence, result in endless suffering and ignorance— whether the ideas are acted out, instigated or sanctioned, whether motivated by greed, anger, or delusion, whether mild, moderate or extreme.[3]

In distinct contrast to the relativistic notions of ethics as related to your caste or place of birth, Patañjali stresses the universal nature of ethical action. In Barbara Stoler Miller's poetic translation of the yamas, we find the principles related to their positive effects:

> When one perseveres in nonviolence, hostility vanishes in
>   its presence.
> When one abides in truthfulness, activity and its fruition
>   are grounded in truth.
> When one abjures stealing, jewels shower down.
> When one observes celibacy, heroic energy accrues.
> When one is without greed, the riddle of rebirth is
>   revealed.[4]

The jewels of insight, wisdom, and compassion are the results of a life lived from a place of nonharming. Patañjali is not offering a magical view of causality where our current actions will help us one day in a future and hopefully better rebirth. Patañjali says nothing about focusing one's attention on past or future lives; instead he asks us to look right here at what's occurring. Korean poet Ko Un agrees:

> Some say they can recall a thousand years
> Some say they have already visited the next thousand years
> On a windy day
> I am waiting for a bus[5]

Ethical action is not based on caste, birth, or rank but on the inherent connection we have with ourselves, each other, the world at large, and the way we see the relationship between our actions and their effects. Positive actions become jewels that trickle down through the web of life, because all of our actions have implications for others.

Our skillful actions can have very positive effects in community and family, among animals and plants, and the reverse is also true; negative actions can undermine others, prevent them from growing to the best of their ability, stunt opportunity, create discord, or encourage bad habits. We do not live in separate and discrete karmic units. Our behavior can significantly alter the course of others' lives. We can help others be free of discontent, and we can also imprison others with our unconscious demands or expectations. Step out of the bubble, out of your car, out of the imprisoning ideas that reinforce alienation and individuality rather than solidarity and cooperation.

All phenomena—living and nonliving—have a life span of their own, however constricted it may be. People should honor the perspectives afforded by such worldspaces. Ultimately this would require a measure of respect for all phenomena, from rocks to humans, from galactic clusters to ecosystems. Movement toward this dramatically nonanthropocentric view, however, first requires development of "world-centrism,"

that is, mutual understanding among humans. Learning to recognize
the influence we have on others and in the entire web of life comes
with responsibility, namely, that we use our ability to reflect on our actions as a means for choosing courses of actions that produce little or
no harm. While we cannot change other people, we can certainly help
people change themselves and wake up to their part in the ongoing
stream of life.

Karma does not connote fate, and yoga does not promote passivity.
Psychological stillness refers to a mind and body receptive to reality
rather than pushing and pulling on life through patterns of attachment and aversion.[6] We are free to pursue whatever reckless and self-
destructive paths we want, and often, in our unconsciousness, we'll
make foolish decisions. The yamas help us make sense of humanity's
relation to the wider world, with the aim of encouraging humankind
to treat both the physical sphere and biosphere with respect, not only
because they have moral status but also because we depend on them
for our very survival. Because of the directness of samādhi , we can no
longer be victims or apathetic observers, and with some good guidance,
compassion begins to rise up to the surface. We take good care of everything we encounter because meeting anything is simply the natural
world meeting the natural world.

Humans and other species don't work without the biosphere. Hence,
the biosphere is "part of" us. How can any "thing" in the phenomenal
world stand apart? We only see the life-forms that we do because of
their difference. Look into the nature of any one thing and you begin
to see where it stretches out, what sustains it, and how it interacts with
other things. There is no separation.

OUTSIDELESSNESS

We can look and look and try to find the bottom and final substance
of things. All we will find are more and more intricate relationships.
Try and find your mind and you will only find relations between names

and forms. In his re-translation of classical Indian mythology, Roberto Calasso succinctly describes the micro and macro scales:

> You can open up any body, any element, with the finest of metal points, you can turn everything inside out and expose all that has been hidden, until matter becomes a whirl of dragonflies. To no end: you will never find so much as a trace, not even the tiniest, of the mind. The banner of its sovereignty is precisely this: its not being there. No one can ever claim to have grasped it. It is like a dazzle on water: you can follow it, but however far you go toward it, it will always move the same distance away.[7]

We can't grasp "thingness" because whatever we see always exists in affinity with something else. Let's not get lost trying to pin meaning to each and every thing we feel or see. And where did we get the idea that our life is a preparation for something else? When we look outside, we try and find reality, and not finding it there, we search inside. If we draw a circle, what is outside is inside, and what is inside is outside. Life is outsideless.[8] Nothing can be excluded. You cannot have an inside without also having an outside. Reality is everywhere; it's the whole thing; even the seas click together in a grand and mysterious moving puzzle. Go deep inside, our yoga practices teach us, go deep into the feelings of inbreathing and exhaling, and suddenly the path leads outside. I look into the nature of the breath, in this very moment, and I'm looking into the nature of nature. All descriptions are secondary.

One participant in life feeds another and lives off another too; the movements of life are a conditioned coming together and coming apart of combinations and permutations, sometimes perfectly sensible and at other moments totally mysterious. Yoga describes this flux, and its practice is devotion to it.

The clouds, moment after moment, unceasingly morph into new forms; and the birch trees in our yard, day after day, expand their canopies wider and with increasing density, and in several months, they will eventually let all those shimmering leaves fall away. The soil loves those fallen leaves. What can live outside such conditions? The executive climbing the ladder, the banker banking on retirement security, the automobile company looking for more and more growth—the human mind always finds itself in the trap of illusion. The greatest illusion is that we can find some kind of permanence outside our own heart. Meanwhile the crab and the honeybee, the ocean currents and the forest fires, evolve and sustain their evolutionary movements without the need for narrative security or metaphysical answers.

Human beings exist within the flux of language and meaning; to deny such activity would overlook what it means to be human. But when we cling to things by creating stories about their permanence, we are lost in a virtual world. The long plains of central Canada and the crystal waters of the Central American coast and the throngs of people on their way to work—we are all at risk unless we think about our interconnections and allow such thinking to change our minds and actions while moving us toward a more sustainable existence. Spirituality is not a blind kind of faith but a complete reorientation of one's attitude. Such a reorientation is the essence of yoga, not as a system or an ancient technology but as a true awakening to the union of all things. This must be the starting point for any form of social, ecological, economic, legal, or psychological change. We must do our best to listen to one another and the pulsing world that sustains us, and to work on behalf of biodiversity itself, not on behalf of our infinite desires and habit energies. It's not just reflection that the spiritual person must cultivate but also the response to the insights arrived at through reflection and the deep commitment to take our practice out into the world. The world is calling out for people like you.

THE ATTITUDE OF SOCIAL ACTIVISTS

For those readers whose path is concerned with public activism, the same rules of perception apply. As activists, we too often preoccupy ourselves with setting up an argument against the other, whether corporation, government, or ideal. Like the secular intellectuals, we easily see all malevolence as being caused by *them*—the system—without understanding how these negative factors also operate within our own minds and bodies. All of us have the capacity for greed, envy, anger, delusion, and so forth, and therein lies the honest reality of how the mind's habits constrict our unfolding. We witness this polarity not only in all the great spiritual traditions but also in the characteristics of our life from day to day. We should be careful if we always approach global problems with the mentality of social engineering, assuming that personal virtue will result from a kind of radical restructuring of society, as opposed to seeing that we *are* the very aspects of society that we want to change. It's too easy to see how the oil refinery is polluting the river in which I swim. But how am I implicated in the action of the refinery? How did I get to the river—in a car? On a bike with rubber tires? Blame doesn't recognize interdependence. If we want to change society and work toward issues like social justice or environmental awareness, we need to understand the inner dimension of change. Personal psychological transformation is key because culture is psychological. Simply performing outer ritual can only go so far, whether in religion or political action. All religious, spiritual, or justice-based practices come down to the personal psychological transformation that helps us think of others and, in doing so, teaches us to become less selfish. Spirituality, psychology, and social change cannot be separated.

Most of our global and personal ills are rooted in problems of perception. Yoga postures are not just about perfecting my body. They are pragmatic ways of working with the stuff of my experience. The way I perceive things and the way I am attached to things determines the way I perceive the world.

If I am caught up in anger, it's not just that I feel a violent constriction in myself; it's not just that I am irritated. An angry state of mind causes the world to appear in a skewed light. An angry person sees the world as threatening. An angry mentality turns the world into an aggressive place. Our internal states imbue the world with those qualities.

When we lock onto a particular mode of perception, we box our world in, in turn boxing in ourselves. Creating an object creates a self. This cuts off the capacity for dialogue and understanding. When we demonize others, we strip them from their complex life and imprison them in the box of *our* ideas.

Habitual modes of perception create radical and sometimes unbridgeable gulfs between ourselves and others. When our mind changes, and when we open up to the complexity of another person, for example, we can open up our hearts and then suddenly our enemies, like the farthest planets, are closer than they have been for thousands of years.

CHAPTER TWELVE

SAMĀDHI IN COMMUNITY

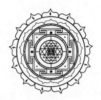

WHILE FOLLOWING THE curving trails alongside the Elbow River in Calgary, Alberta, I stop every few minutes to listen to the rippling sounds of moving water. As I walk along the edge of the shore, I see and hear the currents and undercurrents pulling the river alongside the eroding soil. Seeing and hearing seem one and the same; there is no physical boundary between either the eyes or the ears, the sight of water or its sound. I notice the large steel and copper bridge that crosses the river, and in relation to the movement of water, the bridge seems completely still. Immediately the mind creates two opposing categories: movement and stillness.

I turn right and follow the path up along the bridge that crosses the rushing waters, and I notice the braided copper cables shifting, the wooden planks creaking, and the twisting steel compressing and releasing below each step. In relationship to the water that I can now see between the wooden planks, the bridge is now moving and the waters are still. In relation to the land, the bridge is flowing. The bridge now has the quality of water, the characteristic of flow.

Once I cross the bridge and arrive on dry land, I follow the path that curves left and down toward the shore. I notice that the path is more like an unfinished trail created by humans and dogs and beavers that live in and along the riverbank. The trail itself is changing. From the bridge, the mind associates the trail with solid earth in opposition to the flowing water. When I look up at the bridge from the lower shoreline, it seems rigid and monumental. When I look at the trail from the bridge, it too looks solid and unmoving. But because the trail has been shaped by dogs and humans making their way down to the river, it is in motion; it too has the quality of flow. The river, the bridge, and the trail all flow.

I think about the yoga postures I practiced before the walk and realize that the back bend (bridge pose) also has the quality of water. Animated by the breath, the pose is never complete, as it shifts and moves and flows not just into other postures but also within itself. Likewise my thoughts about the bridge and water, like the movements of the breath, flow unceasingly through the field of awareness. If the mind does not dwell on or stick to any of these thoughts, awareness takes in this sensory experience without holding on to any one thing.

Everything has this quality of flow. Letters and words flow to form one another, and the meaning of these words as I write each one will flow into meaning for you, the reader. A beaver pokes her head out of the stream and then drops into the undercurrent of the river and swims upstream. Though the water rushes downward to the south, the beaver catches the opposite current, only one meter deep, and without effort floats upstream. Our ideas of stillness and movement, liquidity and solidity, appear to be the truth of how things are, but when we quiet the mind and look clearly, there is another truth below our conceptual thoughts, and it's to this reality that yoga orients us.

One of the great delusions of human consciousness lies in the division of things into opposites, categories like "alive" and "dead," for example. "One can see that flow," Patañjali says in the *Yoga-Sūtra*, "is actually a series of discrete events, each corresponding to the merest instant of time in which one form becomes another."[1] Everything is alive, no matter its sophistication: discrete events seamlessly morphing into new forms. How does this happen? Patañjali describes change in this way: "Being delivered into a new form comes about when natural forces overflow."[2]

The bridge, the breath, the trail, the mind—these are all seamless components of the flow we call yoga. In an earlier chapter, Patañjali describes noticing the quality of flow as a significant insight on the path of awakening:

> Focusing with perfect discipline on the succession of moments in time yields insight born of discrimination.
> This insight allows one to tell things apart which, through similarities of origin, feature, or position, had seemed continuous.[3]

Whether in terms of objects in space or moments in time, when we look (vidya) vividly, we gain insight (vicāra) into the flow of life, the way reality happens.

Each and every component that flows through awareness becomes a point of entry into this ancient and always available practice of impeccable attention. Focus the body on the moving waters, focus the belly on the breath, focus the ears on whispering pines—this is the context for practice; this *is* yoga. Similarly, one cannot separate the person, the culture, or the human mind from the landscape that supports its continuity. In an interview in *The Guardian,* writer Annie Proulx describes the relationship in terms of her writing and the characters that inhabit her stories: "For me, the story falls out of a place, its geology and climate, the flora, fauna, prevailing winds, the weather. I am not people-centric, and I'm appalled at what human beings have done to the planet."[4]

THE YAMAS EVERYWHERE

When we settle into the rhythm of breathing and the clarity of sustained awareness, we can let the pernicious thought habits arise and subside. Yet we still need to think and act. The yamas become guidelines for actions where, in the reflective and calm space of the mind, we can discern what actions best express and reinforce the gradual awakening that the yoga path proposes. The purpose of the yamas is primarily social and ecological. The yamas are not necessary in a primal sense. This is a point of great confusion. The purpose of the yamas is to articulate actions that render a life that is flexible, sensitive, and responsible. The yamas are most necessary when we are in relationship with other people, animals, and earth. However, in a more enlightened mode of being, our basic nature is honest, nonviolent, and without the urge to steal or accumulate only for self-benefit. Thus, if we lived authentically, would creating rules of conduct be an absolute necessity? Psychologist James Hillman writes:

> To be in a human world is to live in a world of humans, and in a sense what more occupies our lives than other people? From the beginning we emerge into awareness within a web of human connections that unceasingly engage us until death. It is not merely that man is a social being but that his nature as human implies a life of feeling and encounter with others. Work, art, nature and ideas may take us with them for a while, but soon we are back immersed in "real life"—and real life means simply the human being, ourselves and other people.[5]

Most of us do not spend the day sitting still in formal meditation, nor have we all awakened to our authentic nature. We spend our days in relationship with other people who are also in relationship, and for most of us our relationships have friction. Because we are unique people with sets of preferences and habits, we have to learn how to get along with other people and their preferred ways of being and living and acting. As such we need help being clear, honest, and open in our relationships. A society only gels when it is diverse, and diversity is only possible when we are flexible. How can we make ourselves at home? How and where shall we settle our life?

The sangha of members that practice yoga together is not some throwback, holdover, or relic of a distant and ancient ritual, but a valid form of practice enjoyed together. When our habits and preferences get the better of us, our collective relations begin to erode and we retreat into ourselves with doors shut, blinds drawn, and senses numbed. So the yamas act as a kind of reminder by signaling us, through our lack of harmony with them, that we may be fixed to a particular viewpoint at the expense of good relations. Or they may shed light on the superficiality or imbalance in relationships themselves. The more my actions are motivated by kindness and sensitivity, the deeper these roots grow in my body and in the giant body of our culture. The yamas guide us toward the core issues that need to be engaged in ourselves and in the vast culture at large.

With deep awakening, described by Patañjali as samādhi, there is an inherent understanding of the interconnected nature of reality. Again, samādhi literally means "integration." In samādhi we clearly see the nature of reality and live from that wisdom. However, no matter how cultivated our samādhi or how "big" our awakening, we still have to get along with others. If I wake up in a small town in northern India and then travel to Manhattan, I will have to work my awakening into the fabric of an entirely different cultural context. Perhaps women are treated differently in Manhattan than in my town in northern India. If so, I must put my energy into understanding the cultural background of the present situation. So the precepts are not "rights" and "wrongs" but guidelines for providing a light to see and respond to ever-changing and unpredictable situations. A spontaneous response to life cannot be rehearsed.

The yamas are not a means of deciding that one person is right and another wrong, or one culture chosen and another evil. What is important is maintaining harmony in our relationships as individuals and collectives. The larger our society and the more diverse, the more important the yamas become. Opening our eyes to intolerance, pollution, or racism is not a revelation once and for all. Our answers to life are always going to be human ones, and the value of truth and ethics does not have to come down to some absolute ideal placed high on a pedestal for all to abide by. We don't worship the yamas; we are committed instead to *this* very moment and how we can authentically live life free from fixations and delusion. This means that sometimes we'll be wrong and make mistakes. Even in the confusing and often conflicted life of each and every one of us, we need to stand up for what is important and move through the cynicism and relativism that dominates our ethical discourse.

Awakening to the true nature of our own mind does not presuppose that the yamas will fall neatly into place. I've had numerous sustained experiences of the samādhi articulated by Patañjali followed by periods of confusion and the continuation of unconscious habits. Freedom comes only when we follow our insights through into action. In my own experience I find that living life in accordance with meditative realization is not automatic; it requires continual practice and reflection. I feel like my practice has to do with finding the active edge between realization and action, otherwise the old habit energies continue beneath the surface. The eighth limb of yoga, samādhi, turns back into the first, the yamas. Why? Because awakening to one's true nature does not necessarily give us the power to know what to do or how to understand the context of every situation in every culture. We are not outside culture, and therefore enlightenment is contextual. Our awakening is always set against the backdrop of the culture in which we are participating because culture cannot be erased from our day-to-day life.

So awakening and ethics work in two directions. Awakening refers to the inherent, interconnected matrix that *is* life, of which we are only playing one part without supreme importance. Awakening refers to waking up from a self-centered reality to a world much greater than self-reference. In that awakening process we come to realize the inherent nonseparation of self and other and thus discover in a practical and embodied way an authentic response to the great existential questions of being alive and having to die and then taking what we gain from such contemplation and putting it to work in the world. In the other direction, ethics act as a way to mature our practice by offering us guidelines for waking up. When we live in accord with principles like nonviolence, honesty, nonstealing, using energy wisely, and not accumulating more than we need, we become more closely aligned with others. Every day we wake up and face the world and in every moment we are asked to make ethical choices. What should we do? And, according to yoga, the only way to respond is to become the question, become the situation, resolve opposites by tending to *what is*. Every morning we wake up and come to see that we do not face the world, because the world is always waking up through us.

A literal and purely "commandment" style of ethics alone is not enough to effect awakening. The yamas are an effective aid to practice, but clinging to them as rules can become a hindrance. The yamas are meant to serve the goal of waking up; they are not designed to be adhered to as absolute rules or commandments enforced by some untouchable god or deity. Though sometimes an important course of practice, following the yamas as rules can become another form of attachment, even dogma.

A single experience of samādhi does not mark the end of practice; it is only the beginning of waking up to the world around us, where spontaneous benevolence of the heart replaces self-centered action. With the understanding of the profound kinship we have with all of life, our spiritual life, our psychological and physical existence, and the choices we make create a seamless mode of being in and of the world. Ethics, psychology, and spirituality are seen to be ongoing, evolving, and interdependent, ensuring that our practice does not go stale.

Especially in retreat settings, we can enter into sustained periods of deep silence in which the citta vrttis settle and the clarity of pure awareness comes forth. When students have these very still samādhi experiences, which usually happen when all effort finally relaxes, I always follow through with questions about how they might consider putting their realization into everyday practice. It's not that we need to do something with our insight, but we certainly need to connect the deep internal silence with the outward activities of our lives and the lives of everything else. "Follow this feeling," I tell students. "Know in your bones and stomach and teeth just what letting go feels like. Act from this place."

It's also important not to hold on to profound experiences, either, by making them special or overidentifying with them. Moving beyond the idolatrous tendency in the mind has always been the motivating force of the great yogis of Indian myth because they realized that being stuck in one point of view prevents true flexibility.

In the great Sanskrit epic the Mahabharata, the wise and just King Yudhishthira is accompanied by a stray dog as he takes what is supposed to be a solitary walk into heaven. The King of the Gods stops him immediately and bars his entrance to heaven. Caste law regards dogs, who are considered scavengers, as unclean. They are the animal equivalent of the untouchables. In response to the king's orders to turn around and release the dog, Yudhishthira refuses to enter unless the dog comes too. When he then takes a step forward with the dog, the dog is revealed to be none other than the god Dharma (who is also Yudhishthira's father) in disguise.

Yudhishthira is praised for taking a stand of inclusivity, and the king too should be highly regarded by the reader for allowing the rules to be challenged by including the dog as part of the turning, interconnected cosmos. This story is not a story of one person's stand against a culture but rather the collective awakening that happens when two or more people give up their cherished ways of doing things. Of course caste law continued (and continues) to influence almost every part of Indian life, not excluding matters of birth and rebirth. But this story points to the possibility in the human mind of seeing through fixed constructs of self and culture, fragmented divisions created out of insecurity. The story can also be interpreted intrapsychically in terms of letting the stray dogs of our own mind and bodies come into awareness with no repression or denial.

DEEP ECOLOGY

Perhaps the most significant expression of nondualism in contemporary Western thought is the movement of deep ecology. Deep ecology can be considered the spiritual dimension of the environmental movement. It asks hard questions about issues in an attempt to understand ecological challenges in terms of wider systems, psychology, and the ethical dimensions of various conflicts.

Deep ecology recognizes human beings as a single species in the integrity of the ecosystem or universe, along with all the other numerous species of plants and animals and their interrelationships. This deep ecological awareness is basically spiritual in nature; it recognizes that other forms of life (and thus their well-being) have intrinsic value and inherent worth, regardless of their "usefulness" for people. It further recognizes that human beings are only one particular strand in the web of life and calls for a paradigm shift from anthropocentric to ecocentric. The term "anthropocentric" refers to the way humans regard humanity as center of universe, and "ecocentric" points to the interconnected web we all find ourselves in.

The deep ecology movement calls for changing the way people think and act to include these new spiritual and ethical perspectives, including new attitudes and ways of relating to self, others, animals, and earth. Deep ecology, by definition, begins with causal connections that we've explored as karma; namely, our actions always have effects. The following statement is "The Deep Ecology Platform" by Arne Naess and George Sessions, two ecophilosophers:

(1) The well-being and flourishing of human and nonhuman life on Earth have value in themselves (synonyms: inherent worth, intrinsic value). These values are independent of the usefulness of the nonhuman world for human purposes.

(2) Richness and diversity of life forms contribute to the realization of these values and are values in themselves.

(3) Humans have no right to reduce this richness and diversity except to satisfy vital needs.

(4) Present human interference with the nonhuman world is excessive, and the situation is rapidly worsening.

(5) The flourishing of human life and cultures is compatible with substantial decrease of the human population. The flourishing of nonhuman life requires such a decrease.

(6) Policies must therefore be changed. The changes in policies affect basic economic, technological structures. The resulting state of affairs will be deeply different from the present.

(7) The ideological change is mainly that of appreciating life quality (dwelling in situations of inherent worth) rather than adhering to an increasingly higher standard of living. There will be profound awareness of the differences between big and small.

(8) Those who prescribe to the following points have an obligation directly or indirectly to participate in attempts to implement the necessary changes.[6]

Both yoga and deep ecology have ecocentric, spiritual, and non-dualistic approaches; they both define problems created by ignorance and greed and solve such problems by moving from an anthropocentric orientation to a spiritually based ecocentric approach.[7] Both systems are basically concerned with change and use values and perspectives that are based on spiritual and holistic principles for positive change in paradigms (or worldviews), attitudes, and practices for environmental, forest, and wildlife protection.

One of the reasons that yoga and deep ecology can be so symbiotic is not only their nondual roots or ethical precepts, but that they are both concerned with action and its aftereffects. As we are taught in the Bhagavad Gita, not taking action in times of crisis is a form of violence:

Not by renunciation of action does a person achieve his/her spiritual goals.

For no one, indeed, can ever remain, even for one single moment, unengaged in activity, since everyone is to a certain extent powerless—always forced to act by the constant changes in the basic patterns of nature.

Do your allotted work, for action is better than nonaction. Even the normal functioning of your body cannot continue without action . . . A person doing work without clinging attains the highest goals. This world would fall into ruin if I did not do my work.[8]

MEDITATION

The practice of meditation returns us to this present moment. As we return to the feeling of the breath, the feeling of a body sitting firmly on the ground, as we tune in to the simple sensation of inhaling and exhaling, the mind begins to settle. The power of our objects of fixation begins to settle in with the breath. While the mind may still jump around, it begins to see options of attention that are alternatives to fixation and desire. Instead of being caught by each and every sensation, I can notice the arising and falling away of what appears in awareness.

When I can begin to watch the conditioned patterns of the mind, I make the first step into engagement with the reality of what is right now. If yoga reminds us that spiritual practice is not a system of externally imposed rules and that life is not a ready-made system into which every experience fits neatly, we begin to tune in to life as it presents itself all around us rather than expecting redemption from above. Replacing transcendence with a sense of immanence, everything becomes sacred including all natural phenomena moving through the senses and mind. The waves of conditioning come over me with force, but I am not pulled in their direction. I swivel around on the breath and watch the waves of thought come and go and the stories of myself, like bubbles on waves, rise up and fall back again.

To meditate is not to achieve some perfect state of calm, although that is certainly required in higher states of samādhi. It's also not an attempt to leave the body and mind. Patañjali describes this clearly: "What awareness regards, namely the phenomenal world, embodies the quality of luminosity, activity and inertia; it includes oneself, composed of both elements and the senses; and it is the ground for both sensual experience and liberation."[9]

Sensual experience always occurs through this very body and mind. To interrupt the addictions most of us find ourselves in the midst of, we need begin only by paying attention to something in the present moment other than habit. It could be the breath or the body or even sound. The object is not of crucial importance as long as it is simple. Since the body is always present and likewise the breath, they make perfect objects of meditation. The important point here is that we use sensual experience to cultivate awareness of intimacy, to wake up, to gain insight, to refine wisdom, to act, to be engaged. We are not trying to leave this sensual domain.

The rate at which the world moves through my senses may not slow down, but my reaction to what moves in through the sense doors can be controlled. I cannot change the sounds in the street, but I can relate to them in new ways. I can relate to sound as disturbing, grating, or ir-ritating, or I can follow pleasurable sounds. I do neither. Instead I listen to all sounds with equanimity, allowing them to show up in the wide open field of awareness and also allowing them to pass away. They keep changing; but in the midst of that change I am not pushing nor pull-ing. I allow sound to be sound without turning it into anything else. If your attention span is agitated, the breath will be agitated; if the mind is agitated, the body is agitated; if your eyes are shifting here and there, the universe will be out of balance. Balance and imbalance depend on you—realize this with your whole body, heart, and mind, and your responsibility to practice will become clear.

Saṁsāra is a kind of meaninglessness that occurs when we are so swept away in attachment and aversion that we are lost to the true nature of things and our own true nature as well. We are out of contact, off-line, dissociated. With the mind and body's reactivity temporarily suspended, I'm free to relate to each moment with clarity. Old assumptions and chronic misconceptions fall away; though they may not fall away forever, they begin to appear less and less in a mind trained to keep contact with this moment, this experience, at this time, in this body.

From this moment of nonjudgmental attention, the world opens up as a fresh possibility. The world did not literally open, but rather my perception of it transfigured the world. The sheer presence of clear awareness makes room for possibility. And the possibilities are endless. This is the beginning of intimacy. Enlightenment is the lightening up of habit to make room for experience untainted by unconsciousness. Enlightenment is finally seeing what has been here the whole time—whatever that may be—and then within that space, love breaks through.

Love, in the form of clear, unmediated intimacy, breaks through our life like a sprout pushing through an urban sidewalk. The habits of saṁsāra are the only things that constrain our experience. Over time, the dynamic flow of experience begins to erode the places where clinging dominates. The dynamic flow of life is selfless. Intimacy, in the form of complete interdependence, gives us the sense of being whole and being part of the whole. No separation. Through the aperture of samādhi I am called to move into the world as I continue flowing with the ongoing reciprocity of the natural world without end. When I become aware of my projections rather than being motivated by them, I can distinguish my ideas about experience from the heartbeat of experience itself.

Meditation in light of the yamas gives us a clear direction of what our practice is working toward. Meditation offers a genuine platform for mental health, while the yamas contribute to the social and ecological components of wider well-being. Though terms like "welfare for all beings" do not exist in yoga teachings to the extent that they do in Mahayana literature, the synthesis of meditation and ethics offers the yogin an identical set of practices and, hopefully, outcomes.

The outcome of a solid, responsive, and mature yoga practice is deep intimacy. No amount of psychological ego strengthening can compare with the effect of a self that has seen through its samsaric workings and yields to the groundless grounding of life's pulse. Instantly the body's impermanence has less significance, for life lived in the present moment there is no death. Wittgenstein captures this clearly: "Death is not an event in life, one does not experience death. Our life is endless in the same way our vision is boundless."[10] Every habit, every thought, and each and every feeling comes to be and falls away of its own accord. Every barking dog, when included in awareness and not excluded through the unconscious processes of repression or aversion, finds a brief home in awareness and then morphs into something else just moments later. Each life, even the lives of thoughts and feelings, is so provisional. If life and death are not present in this very inhale and exhalation, we project death into the future. But death, like new life, is an ongoing process of flow happening each and every moment; when we become this flow, we become the intimacy that we call yoga.

ORDINARY SENSITIVITY

Hoping to free ourselves from the difficulties of securing dwindling resources from nature, modern societies tend to overlook the fact that we too are nature. Both self-awareness (which obviously expands the notion of "self" to include our place in the ecosphere) as well as the karmic understanding that our actions always have consequences help form a reorientation in our ways of approaching contemporary forms of duḥkha. Returning to an understanding that human beings *are* nature in every sense means that we must cultivate more small-scale, egalitarian, self-organizing communities in which there is a recognition that the well-being of the human organism is inextricably bound up with the well-being of the natural world upon which and in which we survive.

It's time to recognize that if major shifts do not take place in the authoritarian economic and political systems we continually reinforce, a major ecological catastrophe is unavoidable. Aparigrahā, nonacquisitiveness, reminds us that our rampant consumerism does not bring us happiness, nor does it encourage holistic perception. Consumerism shows us clearly that we are *not* meeting our basic needs. Through our existential hunger we try, and fail, to satisfy our deepest longings. As substitute satisfactions for existential connectedness and basic community, shopping habits remind us all too clearly that a higher material living standard does not equate with contentment (santoṣa) or a better quality of life.

Talk of population control or reestablishing large segments of the world's populations in new territories so as to maintain some of the planet as wild is rightly criticized by ecofeminists for being racist and misunderstanding the interdependence of the third world and industrialized world. Reading the Vedas or any indigenous mythology reminds us that social and ecological balance is tied up with local geography and sustainable agriculture practices. Without a living earth with healthy water and biodiversity, any other social issue becomes irrelevant. Obviously there is no way to seamlessly integrate the vast and complex issues in one overarching manner. But we can begin to see how major social and ecological changes must begin with inner change. If we can't recognize the way our activities and viewpoints support greed and accumulation, it's impossible to respect the nonhuman viewpoint. Unless we act both internally and culturally, no new changes in our ecological viewpoint will last very long.

Human beings need wild nature for balance, respite, and healthy self-reflection. In his description of deep ecology and its inspiration, Arne Naess describes an experience he had as a young boy watching the helpless suffering of an insect where he felt that although the insect was different than him, it was not "radically other":

Such experiences are enough. No definite Buddhist or other cultural phenomena are strictly necessary to start developing the basic attitude expressed, among other ways, by the term the greater Self, and the norm "Self-realization!" This is only to fight the idea that there is something extraordinary and culturally sophisticated involved. Just the ordinary sensitivity of a loving child.[11]

It is in Central Park for Arne Naess, or any other park in any neighborhood, that an urban child can meet the eyes of a squirrel or the patterned movement of a butterfly. The wild can unexpectedly enter the most urban of cities when we have the time and attention to take it in. Of course such attentiveness is only possible when the mind is at ease and creative awareness replaces states of greed and outward desire.

CHAPTER THIRTEEN

FINAL THOUGHTS

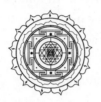

O<small>UR LIVES ARE</small> the live circulation of the elements, and the elements that form us form everything else. When practicing back-bending postures, sitting still in meditation, working through challenging moments of relationships, we do so not as some philosophical approach to practice, but as an expression of nonduality. A yoga instructor practices for her students; we sit in meditation to work with our minds so that we can be clearer with those around us, and we practice prāṇāyāma to learn how to work with the profound energies and states of mind that move through us moment to moment. Nonreactivity takes skill. Once we have the tools to work with habits of mind, body, and culture, we can more skillfully attune to what is happening in the world.

Yet tuning in to what is happening in the world in and around us can be burdensome and difficult at first. It's much easier to coast through our lives in the seeming bliss of ignorance, but the decaying forest ecology and the economically oppressed don't have time to wait for us to change our minds, even when we are beset by apathy or discouragement. In his poem, "The Peace of Wild Things," Wendell Berry describes a response to the world that changes one so completely that freedom is found not by turning away from the world but by tuning in to it fully:

When despair for the world grows in me
and I wake in the night at the least sound
in fear of what my life and my children's lives may be,
I go and lie down where the wood drake
rests in his beauty on the water, and the great heron feeds.
I come into the peace of wild things
who do not tax their lives with forethought
of grief. I come into the presence of still water.
And I feel above me the day-blind stars
waiting with their light. For a time,
I rest in the grace of the world,
and am free.[1]

In the tales of the ascetics who set out on the path of awakening, the landscape, and the forests in particular, plays a vital role in their practice. Turning away from the bustling towns and villages, the comfort of palaces and religious ritual, seekers moved into the dense forests and wandered among the quiet trees and endless paths that meandered through uncharted landscapes. The Buddha recalls his earliest childhood experience playing in the shade under the canopy of a tree. The Buddha was later enlightened under a tree and almost always offered his teachings under the shade of a tree. In the medieval yoga text *Yoga Vasishta*, the narrator describes the natural world with the precision of an ecological poet, making the natural world one of the central characters of the tales. The forest and the human body and imagination are seamless. Trees carry a serenity that is timeless. Trees protect the quiet and breathe along with us.

When you leave your favorite comforts and arrive on the first day of a workshop or retreat, you too are leaving the comfort of what is known and continuing the ancient ritual of meaningful wandering. It's unfortunate that turning to the wild of the natural world is becoming more and more difficult. While the wild spaces of the human mind and body always remain, our forests are disappearing quickly. We need the forests' canopies and the solid trunks of ancient trees in order to practice. We need the intimate assembly of the wild sangha. How else do you define community?

In the Gaia view (of the earth as a living organism), the earth itself is considered a sentient being, and this view would certainly include its tropical forests, which some consider to be the "lungs" of the planet. How can humans survive without the lungs of the earth? My body is made of nonhuman ancestry and is supported entirely by the natural world, and all notions of "me" and "mine" are also contingent on this ongoing process of life including every corner of every forest and waterway. The air that supports us is generated through forests, the forest is nurtured by water, and this air and water give us life. The mind is a forest, the body a forest, the breath a forest.

Tropical forests are the richest and most diverse expressions of life that have evolved on earth. They are complex and fragile ecosystems with webs of interlocking, interdependent relationships between diverse plant and animal species and their nonliving environment. Tropical forests approximate the primeval forest biomass from which they originally evolved and contain more than half of the world's estimated 10 to 100 million species of plants and animals. Worldwide, approximately 1.5 million species are presently recorded. Irreversibly, tropical forests are literally disappearing within our lifetimes. Most tropical forests are too complex and their species too diverse to regenerate themselves from present destructive patterns or to be managed on a sustained-yield basis.

The major cause of tropical forest destruction appears to be overpopulation of humans with current populations over 6 billion and a predicted increase to over 12 billion by 2050. This problem is particularly severe in tropical forest countries where populations double every twenty-five years.[2] This will greatly increase exploitation of the remaining tropical forests and the diversity contained within them, including those forests in protected areas.

If we vow to take great care by meditating on the possible outgrowth of sexual activity, in this case pregnancy and future birth, we must also meditate on the world into which our children are being born. The earth is stressed. What are the ethical ways of dealing with overpopulation? Bill McKibben writes:

> We need to change our habits—really, we need to change our sense of what we want from the world. Do we want enormous homes and enormous cars, all to ourselves? If we do, then we can't deal with global warming. Do we want to keep eating food that travels 1,500 miles to reach our lips? Or can we take the bus or ride a bike to the farmers' market?[3]

Most arguments against population control or restraint in a general sense revolve around placing the human perspective in the foreground. But the forests *are* you and I in every sense. And we don't need a new religion or ideology to save forests and the biosphere. Even at a basic level, it remains difficult for most of us to connect what comes out of our water tap with ethical choice and morality, let alone what comes out of our electrical sockets and exhaust pipes.

Yoga is not a religion in the usual way we define religion as a set of beliefs, rituals, and symbolic vocabulary. Throughout time, yoga has slid between the Hindu, Buddhist, Vedantic, and neo-Vedantic strands of religious and spiritual thought. Yoga is not a belief system requiring specific behaviors based on faith. Patañjali never says that belief alone will save you from suffering; in fact adhering to certain forms of faith can create more suffering.

Yoga is a system of education more than a religion. The system is the continual recognition of the intimacy of our lives. I originally entered this path of practice and teaching because I was angry and anxious and I realized that nothing could quell this depth of anxiety other than stillness. But stillness was impossible to find because the momentum of my discontent was too powerful. My first teacher taught me to sit still and watch each and every breath, and in some ways my practice hasn't strayed too far from that basic instruction. The paths of practice that constitute yoga create such a wide funnel that we first-generation

Western yogis are only beginning to make use of them. We've set the wheel in motion.

When the light of nondual awareness deeply penetrates our perceptions and motives, viewpoints intermingle with breathing and context. This intermingling is a skillful way of being in and of the world because inside and outside, self and other, are seen to be dependent on each other, making them one. Ethics are not just precepts but something one is. Ethics are also not just descriptive of human relationships but also our impact on the natural world. Yoga challenges us to study these relationships through reflection on ourselves (svādyāya) until the reflections release our preoccupations and reveal the infinite continuity of the natural world in us, as us. Yoga did not come from India or Bengal, it's always been here.

In the same way that contemporary hatha yoga practices have been divorced from the ethical and psychological transformations and commitments that such traditions initially required, mainstream culture has largely forgotten what it means to live a good life. In our secular, postmodern world, we've lost contact with, and even distrust, the importance of basic values. Health and well-being are commonplace terms, but only in their more limited sense of physical exercise or lifestyle choices. Yoga is much more than a lifestyle; it's the reality of a life lived in harmony within the entire web of reality. In addressing well-being only in a personal sense and not in terms of a complex web of relations, we have lost more than we may realize. We need alternatives to fame, wealth, personal success, and self-improvement. The security that the banks promise and the fear that everyday media televises reinforce the confusion embedded in our cultural ideas regarding community, balance, and welfare, and though many of us know this in our hearts, we have yet to take the steps that establish a life grounded in gratitude, contentment, and peacemaking. The ground of yoga is the relentless reminder that, originally, there are no seams or flaws.

Perhaps we can begin to tell stories about our lives that are not stories of the past. Perhaps we can imagine a future based on principles that can be experienced directly—not mythic stories of creation and life after death but down-to-earth visions of a life lived sensitive to our surroundings, interested in context. If kindness involves finding out what is good for the other, perhaps our yoga practice and our daily life can come together on this point: What is good for the web as a whole?

Although the basic intimacy of all things is a primary constituent of the way things actually are, and certainly forms *what* we are, this does not mean that yoga has always been interpreted as such. We are all too familiar with the notion of yogis trying to transcend the world and leave the body. In fact, prior to the teachings of Krishnamacharya and his disciples over the last century, we haven't considered the yogin as a householder or been concerned at all with domestic life. This "up and away" attitude toward transcendence is not helpful in a world suffering from self-centeredness and delusion. What we need is a spirituality focused on waking up in this lifetime and expressing the process through benevolent action. That is why this book describes yoga as intimacy and transcendence as immanence; there is nothing to get beyond other than our own fictions. This does not mean we are teasing something new out of the content of Patañjali's *Yoga-Sūtra* or other texts, but rather we are bringing the teaching to bear in this culture, in this time. If some parts of these ancient traditions fall away as we embody their principles and practices at this time, then so be it—we are no longer living in Iron Age India and so we need to put yoga to work in today's complex world.

Every thought, every breath, every cellular movement in this great body is unified. Within this never-ending series of unifications, action is always taking place. Karma is the force of yoga. Effect doesn't follow cause, nor does cause precede effect. They're one, and they move forward in time and they move backward in time. You are the actions of billions of years of beginningless time, and everything we do now goes forward another billion years.

Much like Buddhism's evolution from its Pali origins to its Mahayana framework, yoga must undergo the changes necessary for it to be useful at this time. Trying to find enlightenment by turning away from the world is not only misguided but irresponsible in times of such distress. Our materialistic culture alienates us from our existential basis and as such promotes distraction rather than integration. "But suffering that has not yet arisen can be prevented," says Patañjali in a very optimistic and inspiring tone.[4] It is important for us to allow practice to mature by applying our insights in daily life. Let's not succumb to idealization or metaphysics, and instead focus on the imbalances internally and externally that need our attention and creative energy; otherwise we blindly follow an objectified path.

Psychology and spirituality as well as social and ecological action are all intertwined. Our yogic goals may be inner quietude and stillness, but they need to be put to work on contemporary forms of suffering both ecologically and socially. The organism that is yoga is being restimulated by its move westward, and as it grows roots in this new soil, we must help create the conditions for its emergence by offering to it the reality of our personal, cultural, sexual, ecological, and economic lives. Only then will yoga have something real to offer us.

Acknowledgments

AFTER WRITING MY first book, *The Inner Tradition of Yoga*—a book that focuses on the internal practices and psychophysiology of yoga—I felt the need to continue writing about the practice of yoga by taking the path out into the worlds of culture, ecology, and politics. The yoga path is not just an inward movement that ends within ourselves. If the nondual teachings of yoga have something to offer our culture at this time, it's time that we begin to apply what we practice not just internally in mind and body but also outwardly through our actions in all spheres of life. I hope the descriptions and interpretations herein encourage those on any spiritual path to reconcile the inner and outer aspects of practice so as to see that the two are one and that the discipline of practice has much to offer a world out of balance.

This book has been inspired by the work of David Loy, both through his writing and also through his generosity and quiet support. Over the years, Richard Freeman has offered some essential guidelines for practice through both his formal teaching and also in person; his guidance is always with me. Elaine Jackson reorganized and edited the first draft of the manuscript, and several friends gave helpful feedback: Johanna D'Hondt, Tamara Berger, Jeanine Woodall, and Caroline Mills.

Emily Bower and the team at Shambhala Publications have once again generously supported this project and I appreciate their ongoing feedback and encouragement.

Once again my family has kept my writing process grounded in all the right ways, and their encouragement is so deeply appreciated. The Centre of Gravity Sangha, the spirited and anarchic community of yogins with whom I practice in Toronto, continues to ask difficult questions as we all work to joyfully integrate committed practice and inquiry into our everyday lives.

Appendix

Traditional Aṣṭāṅga Yoga Invocation:
New Translation and Commentary

Aṣṭāṅga Yoga Invocation: Practice Ideals

> I bow to the two lotus feet of the (infinite number of) gu-
> rus that awaken insight into the happiness of pure being,
> which is the refuge and, like the jungle physician, elimi-
> nates the delusion caused by the poisonous herb of saṁsāra
> (conditioned existence, meaninglessness).
>   I prostrate before the sage Patañjali, who has thousands
> of radiant, white heads (as the divine serpent, Ananta) and
> who has, as far as his arms, assumed the form of a human
> holding a conch shell (divine sound, flexible listening),
> a wheel (discus of light, patience, or infinite time) and a
> sword (discrimination). OM

At the beginning of each yoga class at our little hidden center in Toronto, Centre of Gravity Sangha, we put our hands together in front of
the heart, bow once to one another, and chant the above chant. Yoga
practitioners all over the world chant these words daily as a brief ritual
that sets our practice in context. It consists of two verses, the first an acknowledgment of internal lineage and the second paragraph a visualization of the sage Patañjali as the embodiment of our yoga ideals. The first
paragraph comes from the *Yoga Taravali*, a treatise written by the great
Indian philosopher Śaṅkarācārya on the nondual nature of mind, body,
and world. If inside and outside, me and you, my body and this earth are

interdependent, how can I leave anything out? Practice touches everything. Does your practice touch everything and everywhere?

The chant begins with our two palms united in front of the heart, a gentle bow, and a deep inhale. The act of bowing and placing the hands together is a physical act both of humility and interdependence. Though we have two hands, when pressed together, they feel as one.

VANDE GURŪṆĀM̐ CAṚANAVINDE
I bow to the two lotus feet (of the infinite number of) gurus

Bowing is not a common act in our culture. Bowing, literally taking the posture of humility, acknowledgment, and gratefulness, is not a superficial act of religious endeavor but the very heart of our spiritual attitude. In the context of this verse, we are bowing down to something simultaneously universal and particular, not an idol or imagined deity of worship, but the guru in its unlimited manifestations. There is no element in life that is not, in its depth, a teacher. If everything acts as our teacher, practice is everywhere.

The word "guru" comes over into English as gravity. Bowing down to gravity in human form means bowing to someone who understands the law of gravity, one who is unmoved by circumstance. Yet "guru," which we usually translate as "teacher," is pluralized—a rare form of the term. Its pluralization hints at two things: first, the fact that there are many, many teachers that have come before us on this path, which, in essence, is what makes the path recognizable. Second, there are many teachings, for many different kinds of people, and we are bowing down to this spirit of pluralism. Some students practice by following rules and steps, and for many, this is an important phase of practice; but the art of practice really matures when we catch the spirit of the practice and nobody can tell us how that can be done in our everyday, unique, and dazzling lives.

The next sentence twists toward a surprising conclusion. Caraṇavinde are two lotus feet, which are your own lotus feet. Look down; do you think those are "my" feet? Look a little closer and you will see that your very own feet are nothing other than the entire nature of reality presenting itself in this unique configuration we call feet! If you can visualize this, you can imagine that all of the teachers of the past, all of the possible teachings, and every form of potential wisdom that we may derive from this practice all come down to two lotus feet, which already exist in the center of your own heart. Why look elsewhere?

SANDARŚITA SVĀTMASUKHĀVA BODHE
That awaken insight into the happiness of pure being

We are psychologically dominated by two verbs in English: "to be" and "to have." There is a world of difference between the two. Which verb do you most identify with?

The term sukha, the opposite of duḥkha, refers to the sweetness of steady being. No longer caught up in fixation and aversion, we find ourselves awakened (bodhe) to the reality of being free in each and every moment of experience. Imagine doing your chores, your practice, your relationships, with the ease of someone taking a stroll. Bodha (to be awake) or bodhi (to be awakened) are important terms here, because enlightenment in the yoga tradition is described as a process of awakening. Awakening from what? The more we catch ourselves acting out unconscious habits and falling asleep at the wheel of life, the further along we move on the path of awakening, because we shed our habits through an ongoing process of inner renunciation. Yoga returns us to our basic sanity.

NIḤŚREYASE JĀṄGALIKĀYĀMANE
Complete absorption in joy is found through the jungle physician

At the center of our karmic conflicts and tendency toward the known and conservative, is a jungle physician whose skill lies in transmuting repetition into freedom. The jungle here is symbolic of a mind and body entangled in habit energies, misidentifications, and their related symptoms of discontent; the physician is the healer. So again, we find an image of the physician, like guru, as being located inside our own mind and body. A good teacher knows this—he or she will always hand what the student brings right back to them. The teacher is not a friend or a saint but simply one who clarifies, grounds, and assists the students in seeing his or her entanglements as the very path itself. Because the games of the ego are so creative and elusive, we need a teacher and community to help point out not only the path ahead but also the shadows in our own actions and states of mind that we can't always see for ourselves. Maybe someone is pointing these out to you right now: Are you listening?

SAṀSĀRA HĀLĀHALA MOHAŚĀNTYAI
Eliminates the delusion caused by the poisonous herb of
saṁsāra (conditioned existence, meaninglessness)

The entrapments we find ourselves in, the entanglements that put knots in relationship and contractions throughout the body, are all based on having swallowed saṁsāra. In this verse it's said that we have swallowed a poisonous herb (hālāhala) of conditioned existence (saṁsāra), which creates delusion (moha) rather than peace (śānti). The jungle physician assists in the elimination of delusion through the disentanglement of our conditioned existence. In other words, if we are caught in conditioned habits of existence, the jungle physician reminds us that those very habits are the path of yoga itself and it is through our conditioning that we can wake up to unconditioned, unmodified reality.

Instead of compartmentalizing suffering and engineering escape routes, the yogic physician encourages us to give our difficulties a central place in our practice space so we can meet our habits head-on without attachment or aversion. The jungle physician uses the raw truths of be-

ing alive as the path out of suffering so that we find wisdom and freedom in the giving up of our escape strategies. Yoga returns us to present
experience and is not in any way an escape from the unfolding life of
mind, body, and relational existence.

ĀBĀHU PURUṢAKARAṀ
Down to the shoulders he, Patañjali, assumes the form of
. a man

The second part of the chant, beginning with the term "ābāhu," is
a visualization of the sage Patañjali, the attributed author of the *Yoga-
Sūtra*. From the shoulders up, he assumes the form of a man, and from
the shoulders down, he has a stainless white serpent's tail. These two
images—human form above the arms and perfectly stainless below
the shoulders—describe, in essence, the nature of the spiritual life. We
have in all of us the ability to be perfect and stainless, which in figura-
tive terms refers to our innate capacity as humans to wake up, become
ever more compassionate, and live a life free from the turning wheels
of habit. Yet we also have the tendency to shut down, cling, overcom-
pensate, and compulsively identify with thoughts of "I," "me," and
"mine."

As thinking and speaking humans we use language to communi-
cate and interact, to make meaningful sense of our experience, and also
to educate. Yet language and the capacity to conceptualize also get us
into trouble. When we categorize people, abstract our experience, speak
harmfully, or isolate "things," we separate our experience from the complex web out of which we live. We are not neatly defined or segregated
from the relational reality of life. Words can heal, and they can also
harm. States of mind can sow positive seeds or feed negative habit energies. What kind of seeds are you planting?

ṢANKHA CACRĀSI DHĀRIṆAM
Holding a conch shell, a wheel, and a sword

With his or her human hands, Patañjali is holding a conch shell, a wheel, and a sword. These three objects symbolize the nature of enlight-enment—the reality of a person free from lack.

The conch shell represents pure listening and the nature of pure sound. What that means in terms of practical existence is the ability to listen without preference, or what we might call "free listening." Imagine the ability to have such patience that we can listen to others without distraction or aversion even if what they are saying does not correspond to our viewpoint. Listening not only improves relationship immeasurably but also challenges us to be present with and be affected by perspectives that are not necessarily the one we cherish. Relationship is the key to yoga because listening to others always interrupts our favorite projections and indelible beliefs.

The wheel, as a mandala or chakra, represents infinite time. Like listening, time refers to patience. When we are impatient, we are not aware of the time, and when we are patient, time dissolves into itself. When we are out of step with time, there is suffering. Duḥkha is the gap between time and the mind. When we are one with our actions, we are unaware of the time, and suddenly the stream of time and the source of time become one. When we are fully present in every moment, we become time. Time is not something happening to you—you are nothing other than time flowing.

"Asi" is the sword that in some images Patañjali is holding with two hands. It is a sword sharp on two sides and represents a mind so sharp and agile that it cuts through what is real and what is not, what is changing, what causes suffering, and what creates wisdom and compassion. In some traditions both wisdom and compassion are symbolized by a sword or a vajra, a human-held thunderbolt. When the mind becomes sharp and flexible, it is clearly present. This counters the popular myth that yoga stops the thinking process. Rather, the practice of yoga clarifies our thinking processes, because when we are no longer fixated and averse to what arises in awareness, we free up space and mental energy to take swift and appropriate action.

Sahasra śirasaṁ śvetam
He has thousands of radiant, white heads

Blooming from the base of his skull, Patañjali has thousands of white heads, each one radiant and more spectacular than the next. Patañjali is known to be an incarnation Adi Śeṣa who is the first expansion of Vishnu. We prostrate in front of the full expression of reality in symbolic form as a complete reorientation of mind, body, and speech. Bowing, bowing, and more bowing—endless sun salutations to nothing other than everything.

Praṇamāmi Patañjalim
I prostrate to the sage Patañjali

The chant begins with a bow and ends with a bow. We are prostrating not to a belief system or an idol, but rather we are recognizing the qualities of listening, patience, discriminative awareness, and the back and forth movement between waking up from habit and being pulled down by habit as the elements that comprise our spiritual path. Everything is included. You can't ever roll up your yoga mat. Patañjali, both in his *Yoga-Sūtra* and in his image, points us back toward our own self and through that self into the many interconnections in the web of existence that confirm our sense of being who and what we are.

Maturing practice leaves no stone unturned. Like Patañjali's image as both a stainless white serpent and a human being, we have in all of us the capacity to wake up, act honestly, and make choices from a place of compassion; yet, we also have the opposite tendency: to shut down, return to our habitual grooves, and act out of our most unconscious habits.

Not simply a passing gesture, this double motif—opening up yet also shutting down—moves close to the heart of what it means to be human. We all have this paradoxical human and serpent body—the capacity both to wake up and also to shut down; and the back and forth bellowslike movement between the two becomes the work of our spiritual path.

No matter how many times we finish a meal and wash all the dishes, another meal brings more dishes. The practice is never complete. When we give up the notion that practice leads to something, we find a stack of dishes right in front of us. That stack of dishes is our practice. Whether those dishes consist of parenting or back-bending, providing for aging parents or breast-feeding, chopping wood or fixing a tire, this is our practice in this moment. To be fully in each moment, both stillness and action arise side by side. Practice moves back and forth between the two because yoga is nothing other than what is happening right here and right now.

OM

Notes

INTRODUCTION

1. *The Yoga-Sūtra of Patañjali,* trans. Chip Hartranft (Boston: Shambhala Publications, 2003), 2.51.
2. Evan Thompson, *Mind in Life* (Cambridge, Mass.: Harvard University Press, 2007), p. 411.

CHAPTER 1
The Path Unfolds

1. Since we can't locate an accurate description of who Patañjali might have been, I have chosen to alternate between Patañjali as a male and a female figure in order to maintain the mythological sense of Patañjali.
2. Paul Hawken, *Blessed Unrest* (New York: Viking, 2007), p. 71.
3. Ibid., pp. 71–72.
4. *Yoga-Sūtra,* 2.48.
5. *Yoga-Sūtra,* 2.9.

CHAPTER 2
Restraint In Times Of Unrestraint

1. United Nations Development Program, *The Global Dimensions of Human Development,* 1992, pp. 33–34.
2. Ibid., p. 35.
3. Food and Agriculture Organization of the United Nations, *Bread for the World,* 2007.
4. *Fact Sheet* (Boston, Mass.: Oxfam America, 2005).

5. Mahabharata, trans. Christopher Chapple, 13:114, quoted in Christopher Key Chapple, *Non-Violence to Animals, Earth and Self in Asian Tradition* (Albany: SUNY Press, 1993), p. 80.

6. Ramana Maharishi, quoted in Sudhir Kakar, *Moksha* (Paris: Belles Lettres, 1986), p. 49.

7. "Shiva Samhita," trans. Georg Feuerstein, in *Teachings of Yoga* (Boston: Shambhala Publications, 1997), 2.1–5.

8. Wisława Szymborska, "View with a Grain of Sand" in *View With a Grain of Sand*, copyright © 1993 by Wisława Szymborska, English translation by Stanislaw Baranczak and Claire Cavanagh copyright © 1995 by Houghton Mifflin Harcourt Publishing Company, reprinted by permission of the publisher.

CHAPTER 3
Lack

1. Annie Lennox, "We're in This Together," *Resurgence*, January/February 2007, p. 7.

2. *Yoga-Sūtra*, 2.39.

3. Sigmund Freud, "Repression," in *The Standard Edition of the Complete Psychological Works of Sigmund Freud. Volume XIV (1914-1916): On the History of the Psycho-Analytic Movement, Papers on Metapsychology and Other Works* (New York: W.W. Norton, 2000), 141–58.

4. David Loy, personal communication, 2008.

5. David Loy, "Lack and Liberation in Self and Society," a telephone interview with Tom McFarlane, July 2004, www.holosforum.org/davidloy.html.

6. Adam Phillips, *Side Effects* (London: Harper Perennial, 2006), p. 286.

7. David Loy, *Lack and Transcendence* (Atlantic Highlands, N.J.: Humanities Press, 1996), p. 53.

8. Rachel Carson, *Silent Spring* (New York: Houghton Mifflin, 2002), p. 202.

CHAPTER 4
Karma

1. It's not that enlightenment is a step upward. Instead, we might say that the term "enlightenment" refers to what is left when the wanting and distraction in the mind-body process begin to fade. Enlightenment or pure awareness is the innate stability of focus that is always present, always still and clear. Maybe we need to leave behind terms like "enlightenment" if they give us the feeling that we need to strive toward or achieve something that we as of now lack. If we focus on the term "enlightenment" as something to become, we stray further and further from the path, and therefore, it's important to continually look into the beliefs and intentions that motivate our movement on the path of yoga.
2. Thanissaro Bikkhu, "Karma" (Access to Insight, 2000). Transcribed from a file provided by the author.
3. *Yoga-Sūtra*, 2.28.
4. Thoreau, Henry David, *Walden and Civil Disobedience* (New York: W.W. Norton, 1966), p. 101.

CHAPTER 5
Ahimsā

1. Annie Dillard, *For The Time Being* (Middlesex: Viking, 1999) p. 172.
2. Center for Defense Information, *The Defense Monitor*, September 15, 2008, www.cdi.org/weekly.
3. "Peace," *New Internationalist*, April 1, 1999, www.newint.org/features/1999/04/01/.
4. *UN World Food Programme Brochure* (New York: United Nations, 1998).
5. United Nations Development Program, *The Global Dimensions of Human Development*, 2000.

6. Arun Shourie, "Statement at the High Level Segment of the UN Conference on Illicit Trade in Small Arms and Light Weapons in All Its Aspects," New York, July 12, 2001, accessed August 11, 2008, http://arunshourie.voiceofdharma.com/articles/weapons.htm.

7. Data from www.smallarmssurvey.org/files/sas/home/FAQ.html, accessed July 10, 2007.

8. *Illicit Trade in Small Arms* (New York: United Nations, 2001). A UN conference brochure.

9. S. Dasgupta, *A History of Indian Philosophy* (Cambridge, England: Cambridge University Press, 1932), vol. 2, pp. 508–9.

10. Mark Mathew Braunstein, "The Beast in the Belly," *Trumpeter Journal* 7, no. 4 (1990).

11. Barry Holstun Lopez, *Of Wolves and Men* (New York: Charles Scribner's Sons, 1978), p. 98.

12. Gary Snyder, *Back on the Fire* (Emeryville, Calif.: Shoemaker & Hoard, 2007), p. 69.

13. Noam Chomsky, *Power and Terror: Post-9/11 Talks and Interviews*, eds. John Junkerman and Takei Masakazu (New York: Seven Stories Press, 2003), pp. 66–64.

14. Mark Juergensmeyer, "Gandhi vs. Terrorism," *Daedalus*, Winter 2007, p. 33.

15. Ibid.

16. Mohandas Gandhi, *Young India*, August 11, 1920. Quoted in Mark Juergensmeyer, "Gandhi vs. Terrorism," *Daedalus*, Winter 2007, p. 33.

17. Stephen Batchelor, "War or Peace," *Tricycle*, Spring 2002.

18. Ibid.

19. Mohandas Gandhi, "The Message of the Gita," quoted in Ramachandra Krishna Prabhu, *Two Memorable Trials of Mahatma Gandhi* (Ahmadabad: Navajivan Publishing House, 1977), p. 56.

CHAPTER 6
Satya

1. David Loy, personal communication, 2008.

2. Jonathan Porritt, "Edging Closer to Meltdown," *Resurgence,* September/October 2006, p. 34.

3. *Overcoming Human Poverty* (New York: United Nations Development Program, 1998), p. 80. The World Bank data does not include the type of breakdown that the 1998 *Human Development Report* indicates, and while those numbers will of course be different now, they still reveal the stark inequalities in consumption.

4. Stephen Batchelor, *The Practice of Generosity,* quoted from the blog http://quotes.zaadz.com/stephen_batchelor.

5. Leslie Faber, "Lying on the Couch," *The Ways of the Will* (London: Constable, 1966).

6. Leslie Faber, "Lying on the Couch," quoted in Adam Philips, *Promises, Promises* (London: Faber & Faber, 2000), p. 16.

7. *Yoga-Sūtra,* 2.9. My translation.

8. Mark Juergensmeyer, "Gandhi vs. Terrorism," *Daedalus,* Winter 2007, p. 33.

9. Ruth Klüger's story comes from her book, *Weiter Leben, Eine Jugend* (Göttingen, Germany: Wallstein, 1992), quoted in Gernot Bohme, *Ethics in Context* (Cambridge, U.K.: Polity, 2001), p. 76.

10. William Shakespeare, *Hamlet,* ed. G. R. Hibbard. (Oxford, U.K.: Oxford World's Classics, 1987).

11. Julia Butterfly Hill, "Descent from Luna," September 15, 2008, www.circleoflifefoundation.org/julia.php.

12. James Boyd White, *When Words Lose Their Meaning: Constitutions and Reconstitutions of Language, Character, and Community* (Chicago: University of Chicago Press, 1984), p. 20.

13. Teilhard de Chardin, quoted in Annie Dillard, *For the Time Being* (Toronto: Penguin, 1999), p. 93.

14. J. Krishnamurti, *On Nature and the Environment* (San Francisco: HarperSanFrancisco, 1991), p. 100.

CHAPTER 7
Asteya

1. Gary Snyder, "Buddhism and the Coming Revolution," *Earth House Hold* (New York: New Directions, 1969).
2. Mohandas Gandhi, *Yeravda Mandir: Ashram Observances,* trans. Valji Govindji Desai (Ahamadabad: Navajivan Publishing House, 1957), p. xi.
3. Claude Fischer, "Succumbing to Consumerism?" August 2003, www.sociology.berkeley.edu/faculty/fischer.
4. Gandhi, *Yeravda Mandir,* p. 20.
5. Steven M. Houseworth, *The Psychology of Stealing* (Portland: Winter House Books, 2005), p. 22.
6. This translation of Patañjali's *Yoga-Sūtra* 3.26–29 was written during a meditation retreat and study program at Centre of Gravity Sangha in Toronto by the participants in that retreat.

CHAPTER 8
Brahmacarya

1. David Loy, "Awareness Unbound," unpublished essay, 2008.
2. Marion Milner, *On Not Being Able to Paint* (Los Angeles: J. P. Tarcher, 1983), p. 66.
3. "Bishop Demands a 'Better Theology of Sex,'" *Globe and Mail,* March 8, 2007.
4. Karen Armstrong, *A Short History of Myth* (Toronto: Vintage Canada, 2005), p. 44.
5. C. G. Jung, "On Psychic Energy," in *On the Nature of the Psyche* (Princeton, N.J.: Bollingen, 1960), p. 57.
6. Ibid., p. 58.

7. John Muir, *John of the Mountains,* ed. Linnie Marsh Wolfe (Boston: Houghton Mifflin, 1938), p. 400.

CHAPTER 9
Aparigrahā

1. James Daniel, *Aristotle's Nicomachean Ethics,* book 6 (Ann Arbor, Mich.: University Microfilms International, 1977), p. 279.
2. Daniel W. Bromley, *Economic Interests and Institutions* (Oxford: Blackwell, 1989), p. 220.
3. Eleanor Roosevelt, *India and the Awakening East* (New York: Harper and Brothers, 1953), pp. 196–202.
4. Aristotle, quoted in David Loy, *Lack and Transcendence* (Atlantic Highlands, N.J.: Humanities Press, 1996), p. 148.
5. Ralph T. H. Griffith, trans., *Hymns of the Atharva Veda* (Benares: E. J. Lazarus, 1895), p. 75.
6. "Opening Out," interview with Roseanne Harvey in *Ascent,* Autumn 2007, p. 29.
7. Adam Smith, quoted in Julie A. Nelson, *Economics for Humans* (Chicago: University of Chicago Press, 2006), p. 11.
8. I encourage the reader to explore this topic in more detail through the research and writing of Murray Bookchin. See Janet Biehl, ed., *The Murray Bookchin Reader* (London: Cassell, 1997).
9. I do not think that the sole reason for economic inequality is greed, hatred, or confusion. That is just the psychological root of the process. Technological innovation, the loss of manufacturing jobs, and economic policy are the precipitating causes.
10. See Michael Stone, trans., *Yoga-Sūtra* 2.34.
11. Michael Stone, "Conversations with Esther Myers," unpublished communication, 2002.
12. Jean Hardy, *There Is Another World but It Is This One* (London: Quaker Universalist Group, 1988). Pamphlet 12.

13. Warwick Fox, *A Theory of General Ethics: Human Relationships, Nature and the Built Environment* (Cambridge, Mass.: MIT Press, 2007), p. 12.

CHAPTER 10:
Nothing Is Hidden!

1. Richard Freeman, *Yoga Workshop Teacher Training Handbook* (Boulder, Colo.: The Yoga Workshop, 2003).
2. While the articulation of a path helps us cultivate certain skills and insights, simply being on a path does not guarantee awareness since by definition awareness is unconditioned.
3. *Yoga-Sūtra* 1.2. My translation.
4. Bill McKibben, *The End of Nature* (New York: Anchor Books, 1989).
5. This is not a social-constructivist argument, but rather an attempt to see the way humans reduce the natural world with the term "nature." Gary Snyder sums this up quite clearly:

> I must confess I'm getting a bit grumpy about the dumb arguments being put forth by high-paid intellectual types in which they are trying to knock Nature, knock the people who value Nature, and still come out smelling smart and progressive . . . The current use of the "social construction" terminology . . . is based in the logic of European science and the "enlightenment" . . . This socially constructed nature finally has no reality other than the quantification provided by economists and resource managers. This is indeed the ultimate commodification of Nature, done by supposedly advanced theorists, who prove to be simply the high end of the "wise use" movement ("Nature as Seen from Kitkitdizze Is No 'Social Construction,'" *Wild Earth* Winter 1996–97, pp. 8, 9).

6. Trevor Legett ed. and trans. *Śankarcarya on the Yoga-Sūtra* (London: Routledge and Kegan Paul, 1983), p. 110.

7. "Subuniverses" is a term commonly used by William James.

CHAPTER 11
Jewels Shower Down

1. Ian Whicher, "Ethics of Liberation in Patañjali's Yoga," in *Indian Ethics: Classical Traditions and Contemporary Challenges*, ed. Purusottama Bilimoria, Joseph Prabhu, Renuka M. Sharma (Burlington, Vt.: Ashgate Publishing, 2007), p. 161.

2. Ibid., p. 163.

3. Patañjali, "The Path to Realization," in *The Yoga-Sūtra*, trans. Chip Hartranft (Boston: Shambhala Publications, 2003), lines 30–34.

4. Patañjali, *Yoga: Discipline of Freedom*, trans. Barbara Stoler Miller (Berkeley: University of California Press, 1996).

5. Ko Un, *Flowers of a Moment*, trans. Brother Anthony of Taize, Young-Moo Kim, and Gary Gacu (Rochester, N.Y.: Boa Editions, 2006), p. 23.

6. For a detailed description of rāga and dveṣa, see Michael Stone, *The Inner Tradition of Yoga* (Boston: Shambhala Publications, 2008).

7. Roberto Calasso, *Ka: Stories of the Mind and Gods of India* (New York: Vintage Books, 1995), p. 195–6.

8. The term "outsideless" is derived from the work of theologian Donald Cupitt. See his book *Emptiness and Brightness* (Santa Rosa, Calif.: Polebridge Press, 2001) for further clarification.

CHAPTER 12
Samādhi in Community

1. *The Yoga-Sūtra of Patañjali*, trans Chip Hartranft (Boston: Shambhala Publications), 2003. 3.33.

2. Ibid., 3.2.

3. Ibid., 3.53, 3.54.

4. Annie Proulx, interviewed by Aida Edemarian, *The Guardian*, December 11, 2004, quoted in Joyce Carol Oates, "In Rough Country," *The New York Review of Books*, October 23, 2008, p. 41.

5. James Hillman, *Insearch* (New York: Scribner, 1967), p. 55.

6. Arne Naess, *Deep Ecology of Wisdom*, ed. George Sessions (Dordecut, Netherlands: Springer, 2005), p. 44.

7. Whether this was ever considered in the context of Indian culture is an entirely different matter. My thrust here is a contemporary interpretation of Patañjali not rooted in the historical response to his teachings.

8. Bhagavad Gita, my own translation, 3.4–24.

9. *The Yoga-Sūtra of Patañjali*, trans. Chip Hartranft (Boston: Shambhala Publications, 2003), 2.18.

10. Ludwig Wittgenstein, *Notebooks 1914–1916*, trans. and ed. G. E. M. Anscombe (Oxford: Blackwell, 1961), 75, dated 8.7.16.

11. Arne Naess, *Ecology, Community, and Lifestyle* (Cambridge, U.K.: Cambridge University Press, 1991), quoted in Michael Zimmerman, *Contesting Earth's Future* (Berkley: University of California Press, 1994), p. 37.

CHAPTER 13
Final Thoughts

1. Wendell Berry, "The Peace of Wild Things," *The Selected Poems of Wendell Berry* (Washington, D.C.: Counterpoint Press, 1998), p. 30.

2. See www.savetheamazon.org/rainforeststats.htm, September 2008.

3. Bill McKibben, "First, Step Up," www.yesmagazine.org/article.asp ?id=2271.

4. *The Yoga-Sūtra of Patañjali*, trans. Chip Hartraft (Boston: Shambhala Publications, 2003), 2.16.

Credits

Index

About the Author

MICHAEL STONE is a yoga teacher and psychotherapist. He leads the Centre of Gravity Sangha in Toronto, a diverse community of yoga and Buddhist practitoners interested in the intersection of committed practice and daily urban life. Michael's interests revolve around integrating traditional yoga practices in the context of community, where independent study and critical inquiry are encouraged. 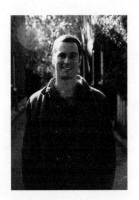 He teaches yoga, meditation, and psychology in academic and clinical settings internationally, and his yoga retreats integrate yoga-posture practice, meditation, and textual study. He is the author of *The Inner Tradition of Yoga* and a forthcoming book of essays, and the editor of a forthcoming anthology on yoga and Buddhism. For more information, visit www.centreofgravity.org.

Also by Michael Stone

The Inner Tradition of Yoga: A Guide to Yoga Philosophy for the Contemporary Practitioner

At the root of the yoga traditon there is a vast and intriguing philosophy that teaches the ethics of nonviolence, patience, honesty, and respect. In this book, Michael Stone provides an in-depth explanation of ancient Indian yogic philosophy along with teachings on how to bring our understanding of yoga theory to deeper levels through our practice on the mat—and through relationships with others.